Assistive Technology
IN THE WORKPLACE

Assistive Technology
IN THE WORKPLACE

Desleigh de Jonge, B.Occ.Thy,
M. Phil. (Occ. Thy), Grad Cert Soc Sci (Health Practice)
Division of Occupational Therapy
School of Health and Rehabilitation Sciences
The University of Queensland
Queensland, Australia

Marcia J. Scherer, PhD, MPH, FACRM
Institute for Matching Person & Technology
Webster, New York;
Associate Professor of Physical Medicine and Rehabilitation
University of Rochester Medical Center
Rochester, New York
Editor, *Disability and Rehabilitation: Assistive Technology*

Sylvia Rodger, B.Occ.Thy, M.Ed.St., PhD
Associate Professor and Head
Division of Occupational Therapy
School of Health and Rehabilitation Sciences
The University of Queensland
Queensland, Australia

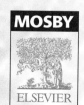

MOSBY
ELSEVIER

Property of Library
Cape Fear Community College
Wilmington, NC

MOSBY
ELSEVIER

11830 Westline Industrial Drive
St. Louis, Missouri 63146

ASSISTIVE TECHNOLOGY IN THE WORKPLACE ISBN 13: 978-0-323-04130-0
ISBN 10: 0-323-04130-2

Notice
Neither the Publisher nor the Authors assume any responsibility for any loss or injury and/or damage to persons or property arising out of or related to any use of the material contained in this book. It is the responsibility of the treating practitioner, relying on independent expertise and knowledge of the patient, to determine the best treatment and method of application for the patient.

ISBN 13: 978-0-323-04130-0
ISBN 10: 0-323-04130-2

Publishing Director: Linda Duncan
Editor: Kathy Falk
Developmental Editor: Melissa Kuster Deutsch
Publishing Services Manager: Patricia Tannian
Project Manager: John Casey
Senior Book Designer: Teresa McBryan

Printed in United States of America

Last digit is the print number: 9 8 7 6 5 4 3 2 1

Preface

AUTHORS' STANCE

For 10 years the first author worked in an assistive technology (AT) information and advisory service for people with disabilities: Independent Living Centre (ILC-Technology) in Queensland. Subsequently, she worked as an AT advisor for the Cerebral Palsy League.

ILC-Technology is staffed by occupational therapists and speech pathologists that provide advice and information to people seeking assistance in identifying suitable AT. A diverse range of people access this service. They vary in their experiences of technology and their familiarity and degree of comfort in utilizing it. The impact of their personal preferences on the type of technology they chose became increasingly evident, and as service providers we became curious as to whether the recommendations made were implemented and, if not, why. We were also interested in whether AT users encountered difficulties in implementing the recommended technology into the workplace and what additional support they needed to do this. Unless the AT users returned to ILC-Technology, we were unable to follow up or find out what eventuated. When funding was made available to undertake research in this field, the first and third authors set out to investigate the experiences of AT users when selecting and using AT in the workplace.

The first author's view of the role of service providers in assisting AT users developed during her time working at the ILC-Technology. This evolved from viewing people with impairments who were "assisted" in finding appropriate technology, to viewing the AT user as a person with unique concerns, opinions, and expectations who consulted with service providers to identify the most suitable technology. This shift from the "impairment model" of people with disabilities to a "social view" of disability was largely precipitated by legislative changes that affected funding processes. Service providers were required to involve consumers in directing the development of ILC-Technology and in reviewing and evaluating service provision. The approach of consumers also changed during this time, as they demanded more control over service provision and were better informed about their rights. Since this was a community service and the consumers accessed the service of their own accord, they were generally well informed about processes and services and able to utilize them to meet their needs. ILC-Technology was also independent of funding sources, so consumers were not tied to these recommendations.

The first and third authors came to this research as occupational therapists and as an AT service provider (first author) who were interested in better understanding the experiences of the AT user and the supports they required to use AT effectively in the workplace. The initial aim was to identify gaps in service provision so that appropriate services could be developed. During the research we began to understand that AT users utilized a range of personal and environmental specific resources and the importance of these. As the research progressed, we became more interested in these resources and their place in supporting the AT user. During the interviews, what the participants said about their use of informal support networks and their limited use of established services often surprised us. After hearing similar sentiments from a number of participants, our understanding of AT users' experience began to develop, and our vision of the range of resources available to them evolved beyond those of AT service providers. We found that instead of trying to fit what they were saying into our worldview, we moved to try and understand what they were saying to expand further what we knew. This mind shift was both seriously challenging, as well as enlightening, and it enabled us to fully appreciate the range and breadth of support these users accessed. The experiences and insights of the second author helped shape our enlightenment into an organized framework that has become this book.

▦ OVERVIEW OF BOOK

This research provided an opportunity to try to understand the experiences of AT users in the workplace, the barriers they come up against, and the support strategies they use to function in the work environment. What we have learned we are sharing with you in the pages that follow. The first three chapters of this book provide a foundation for examining the experiences of AT users. Chapter 1 describes the impact of technology on people with physical disabilities, specifically, on their capacity to acquire and maintain jobs in a competitive work environment, and outlines the nature of specialized technologies used by people with disabilities in the workplace. It details legislation that has supported accommodations for people with physical disabilities and explores issues encountered by people in the workplace. Chapter 2 investigates a number of specific AT models, as well as mainstream models, that can assist service providers to better understand the impact of AT on the user. The strengths and limitations of these models are described with a view to assisting readers to evaluate the models, which have the most potential in equipping service providers to assist AT users identify and use technology effectively.

Chapter 3 examines the process of selecting and using technology from the consumer's perspective. First, it provides an overview of the steps in the process of technology acquisition and use as proposed in the literature. It then draws from these to present a comprehensive understanding of the process AT users undertake when selecting and using technology needs. The second part of Chapter 3 describes the details of the research study undertaken by the authors, which examines AT users' experiences of the process of technology acquisition and use in the workplace.

The results of this research are discussed in depth in Chapters 4 to 8. Chapter 4 examines the first stage of the process of selecting and using technology in the workplace. First, it examines AT users' experiences of identifying the right technology. Based on these experiences, recommendations are provided to enable AT users to identify suitable technology options. The second stage of the process is examined in Chapter 5. After detailing the experiences of AT users in acquiring their technology, recommendations for enabling AT users to retain control over decisions and access adequate funding are provided. Chapter 6 examines the complexities faced by AT users when setting the technology up in the workplace. It then examines how service providers can promote the productivity and inclusion of AT users in the workplace.

Chapter 7 examines the fourth stage of the process of technology acquisition and implementation, namely optimizing technology in the workplace. The first part of this chapter explores the experiences of AT users when using technology to carry out their daily tasks at work. The second part offers service providers a way of understanding the importance of optimizing the use of technology and details strategies that can enable users to take full advantage of their technology. Chapter 8 explores the experiences of AT users in making requests for technology in the workplace and their willingness to advocate for themselves. In addition, their expectations of employers and experience of using supports to facilitate negotiations in the workplace are presented. The nature of the workplace, employers' and co-workers' awareness of issues, and expectations of AT users is then discussed. Finally, the implications of these for professionals providing AT services are examined.

Chapter 9 outlines the importance of evaluation in ensuring AT users are well equipped to be productive members of the workforce and discusses the challenges faced in evaluating the effectiveness of technology in the workplace. It examines the range of stakeholders with a vested interest in AT outcomes and the value of using a consumer-centered approach to evaluating outcomes. The implications of the timing of outcome evaluations are also discussed. Based on the experiences of the AT users described in previous chapters, it outlines the nature of outcomes required to support the effective use of technology in the workplace. Domains of AT outcome evaluation and current measures are then described. Finally, parameters for examining existing outcome measures are provided to assist service providers to select appropriate tools for evaluating AT outcomes.

Desleigh de Jonge, Marcia Scherer, and **Sylvia Rodger**
August 2006

Acknowledgments

We acknowledge with much appreciation the contribution of all the participants in this study—the technology users, co-workers, and employers who gave their valuable time and shared their experiences. The technology users enabled us to gain insights into the obstacles they encountered and the strategies they employed to acquire and use assistive technology in the workplace, and the co-workers and employers have provided us with a deeper understanding of the work environment. The support of the staff of the ILC-Technology, a service of the Independent Living Centre of Queensland, Australia, is also greatly appreciated. We also thank the members of the Reference Group for their invaluable contributions and support of this project.

We also gratefully acknowledge the support of our families, without whom we could not have had the time and personal resources we needed to complete this book.

The funding provided by the [Australian] Commonwealth Department of Health and Family Services through the National Disability Research Grant Program (NDRG) and the Centre of National Research on Disability and Rehabilitation Medicine (CONROD) was crucial in enabling the first and third authors to undertake this research. With much gratitude these funding bodies are acknowledged for their financial support.

About the Authors

Desleigh de Jonge, B.Occ.Thy, M. Phil. (Occ Thy), Grad Cert Soc Sci (Health Practice), is an occupational therapist who began working in the area of assistive technology in 1989 when she was employed by the Independent Living Centre, Queensland, to establish a technology information and assessment service. In the following 10 years, she assisted people with a range of disabilities to identify assistive technologies that could enable them to actively participate in the home and community in education, work, and leisure endeavors. With the support of two research grants, she then investigated the experiences of people with disabilities using technology in the workplace. She currently lectures at the University of Queensland in occupational therapy, where her teaching and research interests center around technology and environmental design for people with disabilities. She has developed undergraduate and postgraduate curricula in technology applications and home modification and design to assist people with disabilities. She is the current President of the Board of the Australian Rehabilitation and Assistive Technology Association (ARATA) and serves on the editorial board of the journal *Disability and Rehabilitation: Assistive Technology.*

Marcia J. Scherer, PhD, MPH, FACRM, is author of the book, *Living in the State of Stuck: How Assistive Technology Impacts the Lives of People with Disabilities,* and the edited volume published by the American Psychological Association titled *Assistive Technology: Matching Device and Consumer for Successful Rehabilitation.* Dr. Scherer has also co-edited the books, *Evaluating, Selecting and Using Appropriate Assistive Technology* and *Psychological Assessment in Medical Rehabilitation.* She is editor of the journal *Disability and Rehabilitation: Assistive Technology* and a Fellow of the American Congress of Rehabilitation Medicine. She is also a Fellow of the American Psychological Association in Rehabilitation Psychology, as well as in Applied Experimental and Engineering Psychology. In addition to directing the Institute for Matching Person & Technology, Dr. Scherer is Associate Professor of Physical Medicine and Rehabilitation, University of Rochester Medical Center.

Sylvia Rodger, B.Occ.Thy, M. Ed. St., PhD, is an occupational therapist with 25 years of experience in occupational therapy as a clinician, academic, and researcher. She is currently Head of Division of Occupational Therapy, School of Health and Rehabilitation Sciences at The University of Queensland. She has worked with children and young people with a range of developmental, motor, and learning difficulties. She has an interest in supporting individuals to participate fully in their occupations and in the use of assistive technology as an enabler of participation. She also has a keen interest in providing consumers with a voice and has advocated for the importance of professionals to learn from clients' experiences. At the time of publication, she had attracted 13 major grants from competitive sources. She has had over 70 national- and international-refereed journal articles published, has authored 2 books and 9 book chapters, and has given over 80 conference presentations and numerous other presentations and workshops. She is on the editorial boards of *Occupational Therapy International* and *Physical and Occupational Therapy in Pediatrics* and reviews for many other journals.

Contents

APPENDIXES

Technology at Work

■ "Computers may well be the most important ally of the individual with a disability in tomorrow's world. Computer technology will bring about environments tailored to individuals, in which the significance of their particular disability is diminished or neutralized." [20]

The technology revolution has had a significant impact on the nature of work environments, jobs available, the tools available to us, and the way we live. Quiet, clean, temperature-controlled workplaces have replaced noisy, dirty work environments. People are now employed in technical, sedentary jobs rather than physically demanding occupations. Computer technology allows an ever-increasing range of tasks to be performed with the press of a button. The quality and quantity of output continues to increase as technology improves. Improved communication has resulted in a network of businesses across the world.

These mainstream developments hold great promise, yet they do not ensure that people with disabilities are able to take their rightful place in the workforce. An increasingly diverse range of specialized technologies has emerged in recent years, designed to enable people with specific impairments to access the mainstream technologies and benefit from these developments. In addition, legislation has been introduced to ensure that technologies and workplace practices do not exclude people with special requirements from these increasingly sophisticated environments. However, many barriers still remain to enabling people with disabilities to be active participants in the workforce, and these require further examination if the promise of technology is to be fully realized. The aim of this chapter is to (1) provide a brief overview of the impact of technology to enable people with physical disabilities to acquire and maintain jobs in a competitive workplace, (2) examine the nature of specialized technologies used by people with disabilities in the workplace, (3) describe legislation that has supported accommodations for people with physical disabilities, and (4) explore issues encountered by people in the workplace.

■ IMPACT OF TECHNOLOGY ADVANCEMENTS ON SOCIETY

The end of the 20th century saw the beginning of the technologic revolution, which began with the development of dedicated devices in isolated research centers and progressively transformed into multifunctioning, computer-based, information systems operating in the broader community.[54] Technologic developments had their beginnings in aerospace research, army intelligence, and university research, and have since found application in homes and businesses around the world.

Technology continues to develop at a rapid pace. The power of computer technology has improved dramatically over the last 2 decades[35] and has become more compact, faster, and cheaper, finding new forms of application.[8,37] Computer systems that once filled a room can now fit in the palm of a hand. Calculations that once took a week by hand, or a day on an early computer, now take milliseconds. Computers were once a major purchase even for large corporations; now, however, they are regular items in household budgets. Technology that once calculated the trajectory of rockets now calculates interest and repayments on home loans or analyzes last month's sales figures.

Even the simplest technologies have changed the way we live. Many repetitive, time-consuming tasks have been eliminated by technology. Time spent performing tasks around the home, such as cooking and washing, has been reduced with the use of specialized machines and devices. The advent of the computer age saw equipment that once required constant supervision being preprogrammed and left to operate itself. Equipment also can be monitored and reprogrammed from another location. The introduction of technology, such as the simple remote control for the television to sophisticated electronic control systems, has resulted in homes becoming increasingly automated. These technologies have given us both greater control and greater flexibility in scheduling tasks. Electronic automation also has afforded us more freedom outside the home. Transactions that were once conducted over the counter at a specified bank during office hours can now be done through an ATM machine anywhere in the world, 24 hours a day, 7 days a week.

Hailed by some as the most significant technologic development to date, the Internet has come of age in the 21st century. This globalization of information provides people with instant access to vast amounts of information. The convergence of telecommunication, computer, and information technology has transformed the way we communicate with other households, services, and businesses.[6] The Internet enables people to communicate from their desktops with others around the world. The ease and speed with which we communicate and interact continues to improve. We now have great flexibility as to when, where, and how we conduct our business.

▩ TECHNOLOGY IN THE WORK ENVIRONMENT

Technologic advances have significantly impacted the work environment. The transition from the industrial to the information age means more people are being employed to manipulate information rather than natural materials or equipment.[1] Many workplaces have moved from manufacturing goods to handling information.[35] Noisy, cluttered, dusty workplaces have been replaced with quiet, clean, temperature-controlled environments filled with computers and other electronic devices. Physically demanding work has given way to technical, sedentary jobs. The computer, which began as an oversized typewriter or calculator, has become a stylish multifunction workstation that can do everything from filing and storing data to complex computations and multimedia presentations. The quality of output from these technologies means that even small businesses with limited expertise can create professional-looking promotional and educational materials.

Computer technologies certainly have changed the physical work environment; at the same time, information technologies have altered the perception that work happens in a specific place and time, in a specific way. Networked computers connect staff, frequently in different locations, providing them with access to common information and programs. The emergence of these networked, collaborative activities and communications offers new opportunities to businesses and employees by increasing mobility beyond the workplace as a specific physical location.[54] E-mail has all but replaced internal memos and phone calls, and has greatly increased international communications. The Internet also provides workplaces with ready access to global businesses, services, and clients, enabling employees to work flexible hours from home or other remote locations. Mobile phones have further extended remote access, enabling people to work while traveling.

TECHNOLOGY FOR PEOPLE WITH DISABILITIES

Because of computerization, people with disabilities now have access to many employment opportunities previously unavailable to them. Through the use of appropriate technology, people with disabilities have been able to compete more equitably with their able-bodied peers for employment.[33,46] For some people, the developments in mainstream technology alone have enabled them to enter the workforce.[51] Others have benefited from devices developed with specific functional impairments in mind.

People with physical impairments, such as weakness or upper limb incoordination, who frequently struggle to access and manipulate paper documents, have been greatly assisted by developments in mainstream technologies. Furthermore, increasingly sophisticated operating interfaces have become progressively more intuitive and user friendly. The move from complicated DOS commands to icon-based menu systems has meant people who are less familiar with technology are able to operate the computer with ease. People with disabilities have also embraced mainstream technologies, such as voice recognition, primarily developed for executives with limited keyboarding skills. Developments such as e-mail, online scheduling, and mobile phones have helped people with physical disabilities as they readily accommodate their functional impairments and increase their workplace effectiveness. Flexibility in where and when work is done has allowed people with long-term illnesses or mobility impairments to vary their work schedules or locations. Mobile phone technology also gives people with disabilities the security and reassurance they need to venture out independently. The Internet has decreased the isolation of individuals with disabilities and has given them greater access to education and employment opportunities.[41] Some argue that the ability to use information technologies has become essential to business survival, and that having access to these technologies is as critical for people with disabilities as being able to access their physical environment.[23]

Advances in mass-market technology also have led to developments in specialized technology for people with disabilities for communication, computer access, and mobility.[35] Specialized technologies have developed in tandem with standard technologies to offer people with disabilities access to all the benefits of computer technology. The capacity of computer technology to accommodate alternative input and output methods has made it possible for people with disabilities to engage in work tasks and participate in the workplace with nondisabled people. The increasing sophistication of computer technology has resulted in specialized technologies becoming more reliable—a critical characteristic for people who depend on these products. As technologies become more compact, devices for people with disabilities become more portable, making community use possible. Furthermore, as technologies develop more style and become more streamlined, people with disabilities are more willing to be seen using them in public.

ASSISTIVE TECHNOLOGIES

Over the last 2 decades, technology has extended the capabilities of and ameliorated difficulties experienced by people with disabilities.[13,20] These specialized technologies are commonly referred to as assistive technologies (AT). More than 20,000 assistive technologies have been developed to enable people with disabilities to be mobile, communicate, control the environment, and participate fully in work or educational settings.[7]

Definitions

Throughout this text, the phrase *mainstream technologies* will be used when discussing technologies that are mass produced and commercially available to the general population. Workplace technologies are mainstream technologies, which are used in the work environment such as computers and telephones. The term *assistive technology* (AT) refers to "any item, piece of equipment, or product system, whether acquired commercially off the shelf, modified, or customized, that is used to increase, maintain, or improve the functional capacities of an individual with a disability" (U.S. PL Section 3.1. Public Law 100-407). AT is designed to work *with* mainstream computer technology, although for many AT must replace mainstream products that cannot accommodate the specialized needs of individuals with disabilities. AT facilitates or enhances the performance of a person by adapting the skills required to perform tasks or enhance existing skills.[13] By overcoming physical difficulties in job performance, people with disabilities are able to explore competitive employment with an increasing range of employment options.[50] AT provides an interface between an individual's disability and the potential opportunities that most people take for granted.

With AT, people with disabilities can connect to the world and extend the range of opportunities available to them.[7] The terms *technology user, AT user,* or *user* will be used synonymously throughout this text to refer to a person with a disability who uses mainstream or AT to carry out work tasks. The terms *service providers* and *AT service providers* will also be used synonymously to refer to people who provide advice or services and includes professionals such as rehabilitation counselors; occupational, physical, and speech-language therapists; clinical, counseling and developmental psychologists; and special educators, as well as rehabilitation engineers, suppliers, and technicians.

▨ NATURE OF WORKPLACE TECHNOLOGIES

People with disabilities use a range of devices to complete work tasks effectively. They may extend the use of mainstream technologies to optimize their performance by using existing features to their full potential. For example, the use of the autocorrect function in Microsoft Word to expand abbreviations helps reduce the number of keystrokes required, as illustrated in Figure 1-1.

Alternatively people may purchase an alternative mainstream technology which they may find easier to use, such as a hands-free phone, a trackball, a graphics pad to replace a standard mouse, or use of voice recognition software. Figure 1-2 illustrates a tracker ball that can be used instead of a conventional mouse.

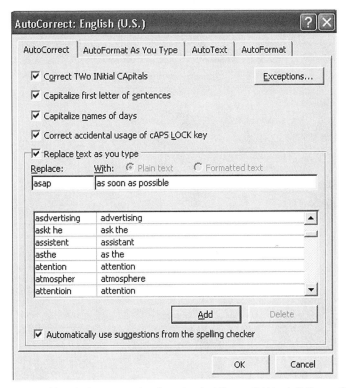

FIGURE 1-1 ▨ Abbreviation expansion function in Microsoft Word. (Microsoft product screen shot reprinted with permission from Microsoft Corporation.)

Sometimes people make adaptations to standard technology (e.g., use a wrist support or a mount for a telephone handset) to position the equipment or themselves to assist in using standard technologies more effectively, as seen in Figure 1-3.

Once standard technologies have been fully exploited, people often explore specialized or assistive technologies. AT devices range from simple low-tech options to sophisticated, high-tech devices.[13] Low-tech options are generally simple and inexpensive and include typing splints or software (e.g., mousekeys) that improve the ability to carry out a task as illustrated in Figure 1-4, *A* and *B*.

High-tech options include expensive, sophisticated, dedicated technologies, such as power wheelchairs, an onscreen keyboard (Figure 1-5, *A*), or a closed-circuit television (CCTV) (Figure 1-5, *B*). These devices are usually highly specialized and designed with a specific group in mind (e.g., people with vision impairments).

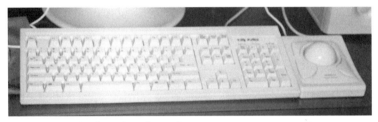

FIGURE 1-2 ■ Trackball used in place of a mouse.

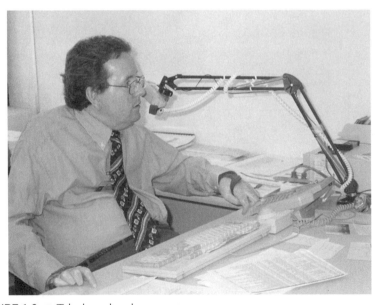

FIGURE 1-3 ■ Telephone handset mount.

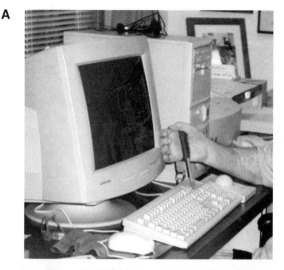

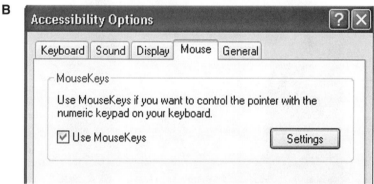

FIGURE 1-4 ■ Low-tech options that improve the ability to carry out a task. **A,** Typing stick. **B,** Mouse keys. (Microsoft product screen shot reprinted with permission from Microsoft Corporation.)

▨ BENEFITS OF ASSISTIVE TECHNOLOGIES

As technology becomes a part of our lives and work tasks change, the workplace becomes more conducive to alternative methods of task completion. AT has had a significant effect on the ability of people with disabilities to participate in society and, in particular, the work environment.[20,32,50] Computer technology has been recognized to have the potential to enhance the quality of life and productivity of people with a range of disabilities, enabling them to achieve more equitable participation in all aspects of community life.[20,43,48] Computer technology also assists in reducing the cost of human caregivers, as well as the cost of secondary conditions.[20] The cost benefits of AT to the community were demonstrated in a comprehensive study conducted by the National Council on Disability (NCD) in the United States,[30] which found people of working age reduced their dependency

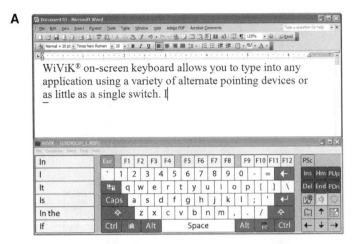

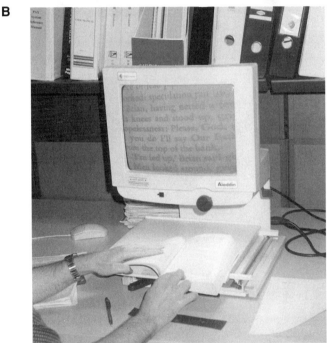

FIGURE 1-5 ■ High-tech options that improve the ability to carry out a task. **A**, Onscreen keyboard. (Microsoft product screen shot reprinted with permission from Microsoft Corporation.) **B**, CCTV.

on their families (62%) or paid assistance (58%) as a result of AT devices. The benefits to people using AT in the workplace were: obtaining employment (67%), working faster (92%), and earning more money (83%).[30] However, the true potential of AT is to enable people with disabilities to be economically independent and valued members of society. AT is often central to the success-ful integration of people with physical disabilities into the workplace.[53]

INTEGRATION OF PEOPLE WITH DISABILITIES

Integrating people with disabilities into the workforce requires understanding current models and definitions of disability, as well as the legislation and poli-cies designed to include and integrate people with disabilities into the work-force. The models used to guide technology application must harmonize with current models of disability. In addition, an understanding of employment disability legislation and accommodation processes in the work context also facilitates effective implementation of technology.

Definition of Disability

Disability has been defined by the World Health Organization (WHO) as "any restriction or inability resulting from a disturbance or loss of bodily or mental function associated with disease, disorder, injury or trauma or other health-related state" (p. 143).[60] In this early definition of disability, the deficit or pro-blem is seen as residing in the person and resulting from a physical, sensory, or mental impairment.

More recently, the WHO definition of disability has been extended to address not only bodily function affected by impairment, but the way in which a disability impacts participation in society and activities at the individual level.[59] This evolution into a more social model of disability has had a significant impact on our view of disability. This new model of disability requires a shift in focus from flaws in the individual to the activity restrictions or barriers created or imposed by society that exclude people from participation. In the Interna-tional Classification of Functioning, Disability, and Health, disability "is conceived as a dynamic interaction between health conditions and contextual factors" (p. 8).[59] A person is considered disabled if they are not able to perform an activity in the manner or within the range considered normal for a human being, with or without such assistance as AT. The standard or norm against which an individual's participation is compared is that of an individual without disability in that particular society.[59] Therefore, the social and environmental context in which the task performance is attempted must be included as part of the cause of disability.

WORKPLACE INCLUSION

Work and employment are important in the process of social inclusion, eco-nomic self-sufficiency, and personal satisfaction for persons with disabilities.[11] Work is regarded as one of the most important ways in which an adult can contribute to and participate in society.[55] Some argue that full community participation is achieved only when an individual is able to enter and maintain community-based employment.[4] Historically, people with disabilities have been excluded from or marginalized in the workplace[5] and, unfortunately, seasonal, part-time, and occasional work is common among people with disabilities.[19]

Disability Legislation Enabling Employment

To ameliorate the underemployment of people with disabilities, many countries have enacted legislative initiatives to mandate that people with disabilities have access to the workforce.[10] To achieve this end, most countries have adopted some form of antidiscrimination legislation.[29] Many countries in the Asia Pacific region, such as Indonesia, Japan, Pakistan, Philippines, India, Sri Lanka, and Thailand, have enacted legislation to protect the rights and ensure the social equality of disabled persons. However, these laws vary widely in terms of how disability is defined, the approach used, and the extent to which they are implemented.[3] The Americans with Disabilities Act of 1990 (ADA) makes provision to ensure that people with mental or physical disabilities are not discriminated against on the basis of disability in the workplace. The ADA prohibits discrimination against any qualified person with a disability, because of the disability; in relation to job application procedures, hiring, and dismissal of employees; training and advancement; and other terms and conditions or privileges of employment.[21] Workplaces with more than 15 employees are required to provide *reasonable accommodation* for an employee's disabilities to enable her to accomplish her work tasks independently. Similarly, in the United Kingdom, the Disability Discrimination Act of 1995 (DDA) provides protection for people with significant (i.e., having long-term or substantial impact) physical, sensory, or mental impairments. This legislation also applies to workplaces with more than 15 employees. Antidiscrimination legislation in Australia (1992), Canada (1985), Europe (2003), and New Zealand (1992), while prohibiting discrimination against people with a wide range of physical and mental impairments, makes no special exemptions for workplaces with limited employees. However, the legislation does acknowledge that accommodations should not create undue burden on the employer.

Workplace Accommodation

One of the most important requirements of the ADA is that employers make reasonable accommodations for the employee with a disability. An accommodation is defined as "any change or adjustment to the job or environment that permits a qualified employee or applicant with a disability to perform the essential functions of the job" (p. 193).[40] An accommodation is considered to be reasonable when it provides equal employment access to a person with a disability so that he or she can perform the essential functions of the job. The employer is obliged to provide such accommodations unless undue hardship results. *Undue hardship* is defined as actions that are "excessively costly, extensive, substantial or disruptive" (p. 194).[40] In the United States, the cost of reasonable accommodations has been found to be, on average, $300 per person.[44] People with disabilities have the right of appeal in many countries if a reasonable accommodation is denied.

Complaints Mechanisms

Complaints regarding discrimination in Australia, Canada, Europe, New Zealand, and the United States are primarily dealt with through arbitration commissions established to deal with grievances related to employment discrimination. Since the inception of the Human Rights and Equal Opportunities Commission in Australia, employment-related complaints have continued to form the largest proportion of complaints made under the DDA.[47] In the Asia Pacific region, most disability legislation relies on the courts to ensure that requirements of the legislation are met.[2] Consequently, enforcement is difficult due to backlogs that, in some cases, may be as long as 10 years. Compounding the problem, people with disabilities frequently lack the time, money, and expertise to fight for their rights.[2] Appropriate legislation that protects the rights of people with disabilities must not be just created and adopted, but effective mechanisms must be put in place to promote and monitor this legislation.

Some argue that the antidiscrimination legislation has had little impact on the employment of people with disabilities. Despite many of the world's economies being stronger in the 1990s than they had been for decades, some feel that the unemployment rate of people with disabilities did not improve significantly.[47,57] In many countries, people with disabilities continue to have a low employment rate.[10] Following an analysis of the employment rate of people with disabilities in the United States between 1991 and 1994, Schall concluded that, along with the growth in the economy, the ADA may have been a factor in the increase of 2.8% in the rates of employment for people with disabilities.[40] However, after examining the complaints filed to the Equal Employment Opportunity Commission between 1992 and 1996, Schall found that people with disabilities were still experiencing discrimination in the workplace, with 28.1% of complaints relating to failure to provide reasonable accommodations.[40] Of concern is that 42% of people with disabilities were unaware of the existence of antidiscrimination legislation.[40]

With antidiscrimination legislation in place to ensure that people with disabilities are not discriminated against in the workplace, Schall questioned the effectiveness of this legislation in actually increasing work opportunities for people with disabilities.[40] A deeper understanding of the barriers people experience and the strategies that have facilitated their integration into the workplace is required if the legislation is to be operationalized. The antidiscrimination legislation is designed to decrease discrimination; however, it is not able to legislate against erroneous and pervasive negative perceptions about people with disabilities.[40] The skills and abilities of people with disabilities are routinely underestimated[36] and employers and coworkers often are not even aware of their discriminatory attitudes and behavior. Despite evidence in the literature of a growing number of services and programs designed to address the integration of people into the workforce, prospective employers remain "hesitant and fearful" (p. 201).[40] Even though many employers agree in principle with the sentiments of the antidiscrimination legislation, they are often reported to feel uncomfortable talking with the person about their requirements and to be ill-equipped to deal with their actual needs.[40] In fact, 58% of people without disabilities interviewed in the Harris Poll in the United States reported that they felt anxious, uncomfortable, or embarrassed in the presence of a person with a disability.[14]

Whereas broad-based discrimination legislation provides a high degree of flexibility for application, it does not provide much certainty or specification about rights and obligations.[47] A dramatic change in policies for the integration of people with disabilities into the workforce has been seen in most countries since the introduction of antidiscrimination legislation. These policies have resulted in programs designed to gain and retain employment. However, they frequently provide limited funding for purchase, hire, or lease of essential equipment (typically AT) or workplace modifications for new employees or existing employees at risk of losing their jobs.[28] In many countries little structure exists to translate antidiscrimination legislation into specific services for the provision of AT advice, information, or resources, despite 66% of human resource personnel in the United States and United Kingdom making equipment-related accommodations.[10]

While a range of policies and programs have been developed, human resource and rehabilitation personnel (70% US; 61% UK) are still calling for onsite consultation or technical assistance for employers.[10] AT holds great potential for empowering people with disabilities to access employment opportunities; however, many obstacles need to be overcome, and resources are required if this potential is to be realized. To date, little is understood of the needs of AT users and how quality outcomes are achieved.

In response to concerns about the availability and use of appropriate technologies by people with disabilities, the Technology-Related Assistance for Individuals with Disabilities Act 1988 (United States) (PL 100-407) was introduced in the USA to create new funding for systems of technology assistance.[20] This Act, later reauthorized in 1998 as the Assistive Technology Act (ATA), is the only established act related specifically to technology acquisition that exists in the world.

The Assistive Technology Act of 2004 (Public Law 108-364) amends the Assistive Technology Act of 1998 to support programs of grants to states to address the assistive technology needs of individuals with disabilities, and for other purposes. It calls for policies related to the use of technology to be reviewed, an assessment of need to be conducted, and funding strategies for technology to be identified. It effected change at a systems level and resulted in projects that provided coordinated, statewide information systems on AT resources for consumers, public and agency personnel, and the development of assessment services.[11,35] Although services created as a result of this Act vary from state to state, they are a critical resource for people with disabilities exploring AT for employment and have contributed to policy development within individual states. Countries, such as Australia, without specific legislation relating to the provision of AT often have services that are fragmented, poorly funded, and have uncertain futures.[48]

▨ TECHNOLOGY ACCOMMODATIONS

For many people with disabilities, successful job placement is dependent on the provision of appropriate modifications and assistive technologies.[50] These modifications are commonly referred to as *workplace accommodations*.

Providing an accommodation can be difficult, as this requires an assessment of whether an accommodation is needed, what type of accommodation is likely to provide the best outcome, finding the specific solution, and implementing and maintaining the accommodation.[18] Placing the needs and preferences of the individual technology user at the center of this process is crucial.[45] The rapid increase in the number and diversity of information technologies available makes this especially relevant to the workplace. Because of the plethora of products now available, this process has become complex, and AT users, employers, and service providers experience increasing difficulty in identifying the optimal solution for the individual and the tasks, and in integrating them into the work environment.[24] While access to information on technology and available resources is considered fundamental to identifying appropriate technology, consumers and service providers alike have consistent difficulty accessing up-to-date technology information and services available.[9,15,20,36,50] Many potential AT users and employers are unsure of their eligibility for services and support programs.[10] Additionally, these services are often scattered and difficult to access.[20,22]

The cost of purchasing and maintaining these technologies is also a concern for users with limited income,[16,20] and employers who are unsure of the benefits[49] are hesitant to outlay the funds necessary to procure devices. Funding is frequently cited as the biggest barrier to AT use, with resources being limited and administratively difficult to obtain.[16,20] Learning to use the technologies also has been identified as critical to confident AT use, but is often overlooked in the process.[16,34,42]

Integrating the technology into the work environment provides even further challenges. In addition to installation of the AT and resolving compatibility issues with existing technologies, ongoing support for the technology and dealing with upgrade requirements are concerns for the AT user.[42] The impact of the AT on the workplace environment and coworkers also is an issue to be considered. The employer is a key person in this process and needs to be actively involved.[31]

Lash and Licenziato[27] reported on an employment training program and followed 24 people with severe disabilities using computers and other technology over a period of 4 years. They found that while computers and technology were valuable accommodations for people with severe disabilities, focusing solely on the technology and the individual was not enough to ensure success. In order to be effective, practicable, and affordable, technology must be evaluated in terms of both the employee and the employer. The investigators emphasized the need to match technology accommodations to employer needs, as well as to the personal preferences of the user.

Many changes occur within the workplace that impact AT use. Although rehabilitation professionals and employment services are pressured to focus on immediate job placement,[27] many would argue that an accommodation should be viewed as an ongoing, dynamic process, rather than requiring a one-off assessment.[24,56]

■ THE WORK ENVIRONMENT

The workplace has already been characterized as an important environment for a sense of productivity and participation. As part of the identity of a person, the work environment affords an important element for the development and maintenance of relationships and friendships that contribute to an individual's feelings of positive self-worth and well-being.[12] Employer and coworker attitudes impact significantly on the quality of the work environment.[58] Participants in the qualitative research undertaken by Westmorland et al.[58] identified the importance of positive attitudes, respect, understanding, clear and open communication, and accessible and flexible work environments as key elements of an ideal workplace. Success in the work environment involves being able to competently carry out work tasks, as well as competence in social skills, which requires having adequate means of communication with coworkers, supervisors, and employers.[61] The human environment and social context of the work environment are important considerations in integrating people into the workplace.

A deeper understanding of the actual experiences of people successfully using technology in the workplace and how they function within the work environment (from the user's perspective) is required to tailor services more effectively to individuals and their unique work environments. The heterogeneity of people, technologies, services, and work environments has contributed to difficulties in measuring the effectiveness of technology in assisting people in the workplace.[17] A greater appreciation of this heterogeneity is required before we can begin to evaluate the effectiveness of technology and support services in enabling people to maintain employment.[17,52]

Barriers to Assistive Technology Use at Work

While technology holds great potential to assist people with disabilities in gaining employment, some argue that this opportunity has been slow to be fully realized.[27,51] "Making technology work on the job for individuals with severe disabilities takes a great deal of hard work in and of itself" (p. 46).[22] Some of the barriers to the integration of AT into the workplace relate to social constructs of work and workers. After years of experience in providing AT services, Smith argues that rigid structures and locations of work, and community attitudes also downplay the productive potential of people with disabilities.[49] Similarly the social structure within the workplace, such as negative employer attitudes and unfounded concerns about the cost and potential difficulties of employing a person with a disability, create an unreceptive work environment.[49]

Even employers who report having positive attitudes toward employing people with disabilities express concern about their ability to communicate with these employees.[26] Being unfamiliar with disabilities and uncertain about antidiscrimination legislation makes employers hesitant to discuss the true needs of the individual.[40] Observations made by Van der Loos et al. in their vocational training facility led them to believe that reasonable accommodations can only be achieved when the consumer and the significant people within the workplace are informed and empowered to drive change in the system.[56]

For many people with disabilities, maintaining employment is dependent on their ability to advocate for themselves.[38] Concerns have been raised that people with disabilities are forced to deal with obstacles in the workplace alone, especially if employers are uncertain of the employee's needs and how to address them. Following a knowledge-based and social skills training program, Rumrill and Garnette found that people with disabilities involved in the program knew their rights and were better able to implement accommodations in the workplace than their untrained counterparts.[38] Despite this knowledge they were not more confident in their ability to advocate for themselves.

Supporting Assistive Technology Use at Work

Gaining employment is often the focus of discussion in the literature; however, maintaining employment is often as difficult for people with disabilities.[39] In fact, Dowler et al. reported only 10% of the inquiries to the Job Accommodation Network were related to new jobs, whereas 83% were related to existing employment situations, with most of these inquiries (79%) related to the purchase of equipment.[18] Rumrill et al. called for more information on people who have been successful in gaining and maintaining employment so that researchers and service providers can learn from them.[39] Inge et al. explored success stories of three people with spinal cord injuries (SCI) using AT in supported employment.[25] They identified a number of areas where support is required to promote successful integration of technology into the workplace, including initial support to find jobs, support to identify possible AT for the workplace, onsite technical support, and ongoing maintenance. Concerns were raised as to whether AT would have been used effectively if this support had not been received.

With the shift to a person-centered paradigm, service providers can learn much from people with disabilities who use technology in the workplace and who have been successful in maintaining employment.[7] To date, however, little research exists on the operational difficulties experienced by people who use AT in the workplace and the impact these have on the user, the employer, and the long-term viability of their employment.

SUMMARY

Advances in technology have had a visible impact on society and, in particular, the workplace. Technology has changed the nature of work available and increased the work opportunities for people with disabilities. Both mainstream and AT developments have extended the capabilities of people with disabilities and enabled them to work alongside their nondisabled peers in competitive employment.

Traditionally people with disabilities have been defined as disabled because of their specific impairments, such as loss of physical function as the result of illness or injury. More recently, the WHO has proposed a social model of disability (ICF), which views disability as an inability to participate in activities, and this may be to the result of a number of factors, such as environment obstacles or the attitudes of coworkers (Figure 1-6).[59] People with disabilities seeking to

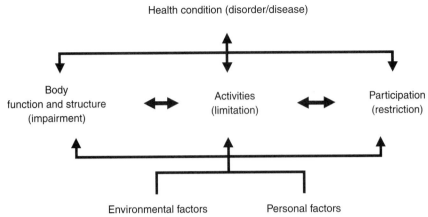

Health condition (disorder/disease)

Body
function and structure
(impairment)

Activities
(limitation)

Participation
(restriction)

Environmental factors   Personal factors

FIGURE 1-6 ▪ ICF model. (From World Health Organization: International classification of function, disability and health: ICF, Geneva, WHO, 2001.)

gain or maintain employment should not be viewed as disabled because they have an impairment, but rather their mode of operating in the work context requires accommodation or adaptation to ensure their continued performance in the work environment.

Antidiscrimination legislation has provided people with disabilities with protection against discrimination. Through this legislation the employer is required to provide reasonable accommodations for the person with a disability. However, the employment rate of people with disabilities and the number of discrimination claims raise questions about the effectiveness of this legislation. Little is known about the barriers to competitive employment experienced by AT users.

Technology-related legislation in the United States has resulted in the development of services for people with disabilities. However, consumers and service providers continue to have difficulty accessing information about technologies and services available. Studies in the post-legislation U.S. environment suggest that a greater appreciation of people's experiences in identifying appropriate AT and integrating it into the workplace will assist in understanding the type of services required and how to make these services accessible to the people who need them.

The literature highlights a range of challenges to integrating AT into the workplace. A deeper understanding of the actual experiences of people successfully using AT in the workplace allows services to be tailored more effectively to individuals and their unique work environments. Although the focus in the literature has been primarily on gaining employment, it is vital that people with disabilities are able to maintain their employment, move to other jobs, and progress in their careers. Many changes occur in the workplace that affect AT use and the long-term viability of employment, which also needs to be better understood. A deeper understanding of the actual experiences of people successfully using technology in the workplace and how they function within the work environment (from the user's perspective) is also required to tailor services more effectively to individuals and their unique work environments. The heterogeneity of people, the technology, services, and work environments has contributed to difficulties in measuring the effectiveness of technology in assisting people in the workplace.[17] A greater appreciation of this heterogeneity is required before we can begin to evaluate the effectiveness of technology and support services in enabling people with a range of technology skills and experience.[17,52]

The role of technology in enabling people with disabilities to be more independent is gaining increased attention. Technologic advances have changed the nature of the workplace and have altered the perception that work happens in a specific place and time, and is carried out in a specific way. For some people with disabilities, developments in mainstream technology alone have been enough to enable them to be part of the workforce; however, the development of specialized technologies has further enabled people with disabilities to compete more equitably with their able-bodied peers for employment.

References

1. Anson DK: *Alternative computer access: a guide to selection*. Philadelphia, FA Davis, 1997.
2. Asia Pacific Human Rights Network: *Rights of the disabled: towards a new UN convention*, 2004. New Delhi, India, South Asia Human Rights Documentation Centre, 2003.
3. Asia Pacific Human Rights Network: *Treating the disabled: rights, not charity*, 2002. Retrieved February 17, 2004, from www.hrdc.net/sahrdc/hrfquarterly/Oct_Dec_2002/Treating.htm.
4. Balandin S, Iacono T: *The impact of socially valid vocabulary of interactions between employees with severe communication impairments and their non-disabled peers* (National Disability Research Agenda No. 1). Canberra, Commonwealth Department of Health and Family Services, 1997.
5. Barnes C, Mercer G, Shakespeare T: *Exploring disability*. Cambridge, UK, Polity Press, 1999.
6. Barson R: *Reasonable adjustment: rights, technology and the workplace*. Paper presented at the Australian Conference on Technology for People with Disabilities, October 9-12, 1995, Adelaide.
7. Bazinet G: Assistive technology, in Karan OC, Greenspan S (eds): *Community rehabilitation services for people with disabilities*. Boston, Butterworth-Heinemann, 1995.
8. Beaver KA, Mann WC: Provider skills for delivering computer access services: an assistive technology team approach, *Technol Disabil* 3(2):109-116, 1994.
9. Brooks NA: Models for understanding rehabilitation and assistive technology, in Gray DB, Quatrano LA, Lieberman ML (eds): *Designing and using assistive technology: the human perspective*. Baltimore, Paul H. Brookes, 1998.
10. Bruyère SM, Erickson WA, Van Looy S: Comparative study of workplace policy and practices contributing to disability non-discrimination. *Rehabil Psychol* 49(1):28-38, 2004.
11. Butterworth J, Kiernan WE: Access to employment for all individuals: legislative, systems and service delivery issues, in Lehr DH, Brown F (eds): *People with disabilities who challenge the system*. Baltimore, Paul H. Brookes, 1996.

12. Chadsey-Rusch J, DeStephano L, O'Reilly L, et al: Use of non-disabled subjects in AAC research: confessions of a research infidel. *Augmentative Alternative Communication* 11:2-5, 1995.
13. Cook A, Hussey S: *Assistive technologies: principles and practice,* ed 2. St. Louis, Mosby, 2002.
14. Covington GA: Cultural and environmental barriers to assistive technology, in Gray DB, Quatrano LA, Lieberman ML (eds): *Designing and using assistive technology: the human perspective.* Baltimore, Paul H. Brookes, 1998.
15. Cowan DM, Turner-Smith AR: The funding agencies' perspective on the provision of electronic Assistive Technology: equipping for life? *Br J Occup Ther* 62:75-79, 1999.
16. Cowan DM, Turner-Smith AR: The user's perspective on the provision of electronic Assistive Technology: equipped for life? *Br J Occup Ther* 62:2-6, 1999.
17. DeRuyter F: Evaluating outcomes in assistive technology: do we understand the commitment? *Assistive Technol* 7:3-16, 1995.
18. Dowler DL, Hirsh AE, Kittle RD, et al: Outcomes of reasonable accommodations in the workplace. *Technol Disabil* 5:345-354, 1996.
19. Fresher-Samways K, Roush SE, Choi K, et al: Perceived quality of life of adults with developmental and other significant disabilities. *Disabil Rehabil* 25(19):1097-1105, 2003.
20. Galvin JC: Assistive technology: federal policy and practice since 1982. *Technol Disabil* 6:3-15, 1997.
21. Golden M: The American Disabilities Act of 1990. *Vocational Rehabil* 3:13-20, 1991.
22. Gradel K: Customer service: what is its place in assistive technology and employment services? *Vocational Rehabil* 3:41-54, 1991.
23. Hammel JM, Smith RO: The development of technology competencies and training guidelines for occupational therapists. *Am J Occup Ther* 47(11):970-979, 1993.
24. Hammel JM, Symons J: Evaluating for reasonable accommodation: a team approach. *J Prevention Assessment Rehabil* 3(4):12-21, 1993.
25. Inge KJ, Wehman P, Strobel W, et al: Supported employment and assistive technology for persons with spinal cord injury: three illustrations of successful work supports. *J Vocational Rehabil* 10:141-152, 1998.
26. Kregel J, Tomiyasu Y: Employers' attitudes toward workers with disabilities: effect of the Americans with Disabilities Act. *J Vocational Rehabil* 4(3):165-173, 1994.
27. Lash M, Licenziato V: Career transitions for people with severe physical disabilities: integrating technology and psychosocial skills and accommodations. *Work* 5:85-98, 1995.
28. Lunt N, Thornton P: Employment policies for disabled people. Moorfoot, England, Research Management Branch, Employment Dept., 1993.
29. Lunt N, Thornton P (eds): Researching disability employment policies. Leeds, England, The Disability Press, 1997.
30. National Council of Disability: Study on the financing of assistive technology devices and services for individuals with disabilities. Washington, DC, National Council on Disability, 1993.
31. Nochajski SM, Oddo CR: Technology in the workplace, in Mann WC, Lane JP (eds): *Assistive technology for people with disabilities,* ed 2. Bethesda, MD, AOTA, 1995.
32. O'Day BL, Corcoran PJ: Assistive technology: problems and policy alternatives. *Arch Phys Med Rehabil* 75:1165-1169, 1994.
33. Pell SB, Gillies RM, Carss M: Relationship between use of technology and employment rates for people with physical disabilities in Australia: publication for education and training programmes. *Disabil Rehabil* 19(8):332-338, 1997.

34. Pell SB, Gillies RM, Carss M: Use of technology by people with physical disabilities in Australia. *Disabil Rehabil* 21(2):56-60, 1999.
35. Post KM: The promise of assistive technology. *Am J Occup Ther* 47(11):965-967, 1993.
36. Robinson JE: Access to employment for people with disabilities: findings of a consumer-led project. *Disabil Rehabil* 22(5):246-253, 2000.
37. Rohl JS: Technology directions and their impact on the way we work, 1998. Retrieved September 2000, from www.doplar.wa.gov.au/w&f/wfcr/rohl.html.
38. Rumrill PD, Garnette M: Career adjustment via reasonable accommodations: the effects of an employee-empowerment intervention for people with disabilities. *J Prevention Assessment Rehabil* 9:57-64, 1997.
39. Rumrill PD, Steffen J, Kaleta D, et al: Job placement interventions for people with multiple sclerosis. *Work* 6:167-175, 1996.
40. Schall CM: The American Disabilities Act: are we keeping our promise? An analysis of the effect of the ADA on the employment of persons with disabilities. *J Vocational Rehabil* 10:191-203, 1998.
41. Scherer MJ: Connecting to learn: educational and assistive technology for people with disabilities, Washington, DC, American Psychological Association (APA) Books, 2004.
42. Scherer MJ: Living in a state of stuck: how assistive technology impacts the lives of people with disabilities, ed 4. Cambridge, MA, Brookline Books, 2005.
43. Scherer MJ: The impact of assistive technology on the lives of people with disabilities, in Gray DB, Quatrano LA, Lieberman ML (eds): Designing and using assistive technology: the human perspective. Baltimore, Paul H. Brookes, 1998.
44. Scherer MJ, McKee B: What employees want to know about assistive technology in the workplace. *SHHH J* 14(1):23-27, 1993.
45. Scherer MJ, Vitaliti LT: Functional approach to technological factors and their assessment in rehabilitation, in Dittmar SS, Gresham GE (eds): Functional assessment and outcome measures for the health rehabilitation professional. Gaithersburg, MD, Aspen, 1997.
46. Schneider M: Achieving greater independence through assistive technology, job accommodation and supported employment. *J Vocational Rehabil* 12:159-164, 1999.
47. Sidoti C: *The DDA and employment of people with a disability*, 1998. Retrieved October 10, 2004, from www.hreoc.gov.au//disability_rights/speeches/1998/employment_98.html.
48. Smith G: *Computers and the employment of people with a severe physical disability*. Paper presented at the Australian Conference on Technology for People with Disabilities, Adelaide, South Australia, October 9-12, 1995.
49. Smith G: *The impact of speech recognition on people with disabilities* (National Disability Research Agenda No. 1), Canberra, Australia, Commonwealth Department of Health and Family Services, 1997.
50. Sowers JA: Adaptive environments in the workplace, in Flippo KF, Inge KJ, Barcus JM (eds): *Assistive technology: a resource for school, work and community*. Baltimore, Paul H. Brookes, 1995.
51. Sowers JA: Employment for persons with physical disabilities and related technology. *Vocational Rehabil* 3:55-64, 1991.
52. Spencer JC: Tools or baggage? Alternative meanings of assistive technology, in Gray DB, Quatrano LA, Lieberman ML (eds): *Designing and using assistive technology: the human perspective*. Baltimore, Paul H. Brookes, 1998.
53. Steinfeld E, Angelo J: Adaptive work placement: a "horizontal" model. *Technol Disabil* 1(4):1-10, 1992.

54. Stephanidis C, Emiliani PL: "Connecting" to the information society: a European perspective. *Technol Disabil* 10:21-44, 1999.
55. Storey K, Ezell H, Lengyel L: Communication strategies for increasing the integration of persons in supported employment: a review. *Am J Speech-Language Pathology* 4:45-54, 1995.
56. Van der Loos HFM, Machiel HF, Hammel J: Engineering reasonable accommodation: the delivery and use of assistive technology in a vocational training program. *Technol Disabil* 5:371-382, 1996.
57. Wehman P: Work, employment and disability: meeting the challenge. *J Vocational Rehabil* 11(1):1-3, 1998.
58. Westmorland MG, Zeytinoglu I, Pringle P, et al: The elements of a positive workplace environment: implications for persons with disabilities. *J Prevention Assessment Rehabil* 10:109-117, 1998.
59. World Health Organization: International classification of function, disability and health: ICF, Geneva, WHO, 2001.
60. World Health Organization: The international classification of impairments, disabilities and handicaps (ICIDH). Geneva, WHO, 1980.
61. Yvislaker M, Urbanczyk B, Feeney TJ: Social skills following traumatic brain injury. *Sem Speech Language* 13:308-319, 1992.

CHAPTER 2

Review of the Development of Assistive Technology Models

■ "Technology is the answer, but that's not the question."[42]

T his chapter investigates a number of specific assistive technology (AT) models as well as mainstream models that can assist service providers to better understand the impact of AT on the user. Specifically the rehabilitation model, the needs-based model, the human activity assistive technology (HAAT) model, and the matching person and technology (MPT) model are described. In addition, mainstream models, such as human-centered design and attributional models, are discussed in terms of their application to understanding AT users. The strengths and limitations of these models are described with a view to assisting readers to evaluate the models that have the most potential in equipping service providers to assist AT users identify and use technology effectively.

Models, conceptual or procedural, provide a framework for thinking and practice.[39] Conceptual models present an overview of issues of a concept or object, providing an understanding of the elements involved and how they interact. Procedural models, on the other hand, detail the process for addressing issues. For example, if you were planning a trip, a map (a conceptual representation) could tell you where things are and how they relate to each other spatially, whereas a travel schedule (a procedural plan) provides you with details of the times and routes of travel. Some models are inherently conceptual in nature, leaving clinicians to develop their own framework for implementation, whereas others are primarily procedural and may or may not detail their conceptual framework. A number of models incorporate both elements, as they provide a conceptual framework and then detail how it should be operationalized. Both types of models are needed to function effectively. We need to know where we are headed and how our various landmarks and stopovers relate to each other; we need a plan of action to ensure we get to see all the important sights and arrive at our destination efficiently.

Over the years, AT practice has drawn knowledge from a number of models. Initially, AT practice drew from traditional health models, such as the rehabilitation model. More recently, AT practice has developed its own frameworks to address the complexities involved with technology selection and application. This chapter will (1) describe the evolution of models related to technology application, (2) investigate how they impact on the nature of services delivered, and (3) examine the relevance and integrity of these models in light of recent politicosociocultural trends, specifically the shift toward consumer-driven services. The models will be described in terms of their scope of concern, AT user involvement, issue or problem definition, service provider role, assessment strategies used, interventions prescribed, evaluation of technology considered, and finally, the outcomes that are the focus of the model.

Whether we are conscious of the conceptual models with which we work, each of us holds a view of people and an understanding of the cause and impact of impairment or disability. These views define our scope of concern and the nature of the services we offer. They dictate how we work with AT users, determine their needs, and the focus of our interventions. Some service providers may not be aware of the models that color their thinking and guide their practice, but this does not mean that they do not have them. Concepts are embedded in their thinking. Their practice feels largely intuitive to them.[39] These providers select and apply assessments and interventions, unaware of the beliefs and attitudes that direct their actions. Without a clearly identified model to define the scope of practice and provide a systematic approach, practice is reliant on trial and error as well as personal experience.[21] Service providers who are not conscious of their practice framework may find themselves at odds with consumers or other service providers without understanding why. They may also find it more difficult to recognize and respond to conceptual changes and new knowledge in an area of practice.

Practitioners who consciously seek conceptual frameworks to make sense of their clinical experiences may align themselves with a particular model or number of models. These service providers use models to define clearly and articulate their scope of concern and assist them in understanding issues and the complex interplay of factors. By identifying and naming pertinent factors, conceptual models make it possible for practitioners to address all the relevant issues and to select and target interventions appropriately. Models help them to translate intuitive ideas and hunches into concepts that can be articulated, discussed, and reflected upon.[39] Starting with models, the service provider and the field of practice can continue to grow and develop as new knowledge and understandings come to light.

Throughout this chapter, the case study of Steven will be used to illustrate the impact different models have on the range and nature of services offered. The way practitioners view Steven, relate to him, and define his needs reveals the model of practice from which they work. Take time to reflect on this case and write down your thoughts before continuing. As you read through this chapter you may recognize aspects of models evident in your approach to Steven, and come to appreciate the impact of your current conceptualizations regarding the nature of the services you provide, the procedures you use, and the subsequent outcomes for Steven. Take this opportunity to reflect on contemporary views of disability and client-centered practice, and how well they are reflected in your current practice.

CASE STUDY: STEVEN

Steven is a 28-year-old man who has been hospitalized with a fracture of C6/7 vertebrae, following an accident during an extreme sports competition. Prior to the injury Steven was a very active man. He has a degree in physical education and teaches at a high school. He has not had a lot of experience with computers and does not consider himself to be computer literate. He is close to returning home and interested in exploring how technology can assist him. How would you assist Steven in identifying his technology needs?

Traditionally, assistive technology needs were addressed within the medical system where service providers operated from the rehabilitation model. As AT service delivery developed and expanded into the community, models were devised to direct practice in various settings. Needs-based models evolved to enable practitioners to identify the individual's specific goals and use a systematic process for selecting technology. In the last decade, contemporary AT models have been created that identify the multiple factors involved in AT use, and how these factors interact[25] and promote a systematic approach to service delivery. AT models have continued to evolve in response to an increased understanding of issues and factors underlying AT use, as well as the trends in society, such as the shift to a social model of disability and consumer-driven services. By examining the evolution of AT models, we can examine the impact of models on our practice, how and why practice has changed, and how well models reflect current politicosociocultural trends. In addition, a review of some contemporary models will identify similarities and the unique contribution each has made to our understanding of technology selection and use.

■ REHABILITATION FOUNDATION OF ASSISTIVE TECHNOLOGY PRACTICE

AT services have grown out of the rehabilitation paradigm, and many current assessment and intervention practices are rooted in this model. Rehabilitation is described as "a process of restoring an individual's capacity to participate in functional activities when the capacity has been altered or limited by a physical or mental impairment" (p. 536).[46] This framework is based on a solid understanding of the structure and function of the human body and the impact of injury and disease. The rehabilitation paradigm, as we know it today, began in earnest after World War II (WWII) when large numbers of wounded soldiers required repatriation. Much of the early writing in rehabilitation suggested that programs focused on restoring lost function.[46] When restoration of function was not possible, retraining was provided in an effort to regain as much independence as possible. Compensation strategies were then initiated when it was clear that full function could not be regained. In addition, assistive devices were used at this time when loss of limbs or permanent injuries necessitated the fabrication of prostheses and specialized equipment.

The rehabilitation paradigm has evolved slowly over the years in response to social changes. However, the focus of this paradigm on body functions and structure has had an enduring impact on the way people with disabilities are viewed and their needs defined. People are viewed as human organisms consisting of a series of systems, underlying structures, and functions common to all humans. Generally, rehabilitation professionals define their scope of concern or responsibilities in terms of a body system; for example, physiotherapists are concerned with neuromuscular function, psychologists address cognitive functions, and speech pathologists focus on voice and speech functions. Alternatively some professions have focused on the functional manifestations of structural changes resulting from injury or disease, such as occupational therapists who focus on the person's ability to function in daily activities. In this model, *impairment* is defined as the "loss or abnormality of psychological, physiological or anatomical structure or function" (p. 47),[57] whereas *disability* is viewed as a restriction or lack of ability to perform an activity in a manner or within the range considered normal.[46] Assessment in this model usually focuses on identifying specific symptoms and signs of abnormality and determining the person's capacities in relation to areas of function, such as neuromuscular, cognitive, or cardiovascular function. Interventions involve the combined and coordinated use of medical, social, educational, and vocational measures to train or retrain an individual to the highest possible levels of function.[57] These interventions include remediation activities to restore function, compensatory methods to complete actions or tasks and assistive devices, and environmental adaptations to accommodate lost function.

The focus of the rehabilitation model is to achieve maximum skills and independence, with the potential for regaining independence being contingent on the person's level of motivation. In this model, service providers are seen as experts who bring specialist knowledge about the physiology and pathology of impairment and appropriate remediation and compensation strategies.[16] Service providers instruct clients on how to regain lost function or advise them on suitable compensatory techniques, assistive devices, or environmental adaptations. With its strong scientific basis, the rehabilitation model has a keen interest in the potential of technology for investigating pathology and injury, and replacing injured parts (e.g., joint replacements). The potential of technology for retraining and skill development, such as developing cognitive skills using computer games or correcting postural deformities with seating inserts, has also been explored. In addition, many assistive devices have been developed to accommodate specific loss of function (e.g., manual wheelchairs for people with paraplegia and powered wheelchairs for people with quadriplegia). In the rehabilitation model, AT devices are frequently prescribed by first identifying the person's impairment to determine the type of device they require and then assessing whether they have the capacity to operate the device. The person's physical dimensions are then measured to identify the size and strength requirements needed to use the technology. The outcome sought by all these interventions is for the person to return home and to be as independent as possible. Consequently, outcome measures focus on the person's level of independence and function believed to underpin independence.

Working with Steven Using the Rehabilitation Model

In light of the previous description of the rehabilitation model, we now return to consider the implications of using this model in addressing Steven's technology needs. Some questions which arise include the following:

- How would a service provider using a rehabilitation framework view him?
- How would a service provider define Steven's needs?
- What assessment processes would he experience?
- What interventions or services would be available to him?
- How would the service provider relate to him?
- How would the technology be selected and applied?

The amount of scientific knowledge underlying the rehabilitation model is extensive. Consequently, Steven would receive the very best medical care, resulting in him retaining as much function as possible after his injury. Each service provider would take responsibility for body systems within their scope of concern and ensure that he regained maximum capacity and received training in compensatory techniques as required. Steven would frequently be identified by his impairment, that is, as a person with a spinal injury and, in some cases, as having a C6/7 level of injury and be provided services accordingly. The system would be largely focused on his physical rehabilitation and would work to help him "accept his disability"[16] (Table 2-1). Lack of expected progress would be attributed to Steven's lack of motivation, and any emotional responses to his injury that significantly impeded his progress would be referred to an appropriate specialist. Assessments would focus on defining his loss of function. Steven would experience repeated assessment of his physical and functional

TABLE 2-1

Defining Steven's AT Requirements Using the Rehabilitation Model

DEFINED STRENGTHS	DEFINED NEEDS	TECHNOLOGY REQUIREMENTS/ CHARACTERISTICS
Good upper limb strength	Limited hand function	Manual wheelchair with coated rims or power-assist push rims or power wheelchair
Cognition is intact	Inability to propel a standard wheelchair independently	
		Hand/finger splints
	Intermittent skin breakdown	Pressure cushions
		Transfer board/Hoyer lift

capacity. Goals would be set for maximum function, and intervention would consist of exercises, skill-building activities, and retraining in activities of daily living considered normal (e.g., all adults are expected to be independent in bathing). Steven would rely on the expertise of the service providers who would advise him on appropriate activities to regain capacities and skills and suitable equipment. Because he has a spinal injury and is not able to regain his ability to walk, he would be prescribed a wheelchair defined by his capacity to propel, his weight, size, and propensity for pressure sores. Other devices also would be recommended based on his diagnosis (e.g., reachers, environmental controls, remote control devices).[28] Steven also would be advised to modify his home environment to accommodate his wheelchair (e.g., put in ramps, raise his desk, and clear circulation spaces). Table 2-1 outlines Steven's technology needs as identified by the rehabilitation model. If technology is made available to him in rehabilitation, he would most likely be encouraged to build computer skills in preparation for returning to a less physically demanding job. The nature of technology explored with Steven would depend on the time available in hospital, the availability of personnel with suitable expertise in technology, the scope of the services available to address domestic, leisure, and work aspects of his life, and the funding available for purchasing equipment and services. Steven's ability to perform daily activities independently would determine the success of the interventions; however, in lieu of effective outcome measurement tools, the professional's judgment could be frequently called on to determine if Steven required further follow-up after discharge.

Implications of the Rehabilitation Model for Assistive Technology Users

As noted previously, the extensive science underlying the rehabilitation model has enabled many people with disabilities to retain high levels of function after injury. The rehabilitation model grew out of the medical model that was responsible originally for treating sick people who were dependent on health professionals to locate the cause of the illness and treat it. Consequently, this model uses a medical or individual model of disability where disablement is viewed as a personal problem, directly caused by disease, trauma, or health conditions, and requires medical care provided by professionals in the form of individual treatment.[3] Focusing on the presenting injury and impaired systems can often result in people being fragmented and feeling dehumanized. The medicalization of disability also has viewed impairment as a personal tragedy requiring "adjustment."[33] This emphasis on the person's deficits can negatively impact the person's view of him- or herself,[10] and place him or her at risk of focusing on the losses rather than exploring the future.

Assessments and treatment protocols in the rehabilitation model do not allow the practitioner to develop an understanding of the real person, what they do, and with whom they live. This lack of understanding makes it difficult to attend to the unique life experiences of the person. An emphasis on regaining function and independence in daily living activities often leaves little time for personal goals to be formulated or addressed. Furthermore, goals set for maximum function may not accurately reflect the strength and movement requirements for an individual and may overestimate or underestimate the capacities they require to re-engage in life. Although we have charts that detail the average grip strength for people of varying ages, little is known about the minimum strength requirements of everyday tasks. The strength requirements of an office worker would differ greatly from the strength requirements of a fitter and turner. Much of what is defined as "normal" is also highly influenced by personal values. Whereas the clinician may value independence in showering, the client may prefer to receive assistance in self-care and invest his or her valuable time and energy in work tasks. When a person presents with a physical impairment, his social and emotional needs are often overlooked unless they have a significant effect on progress. Failure to achieve predetermined outcomes is attributed frequently to the person's lack of motivation, rather than the goals and interventions being irrelevant to the individual.

With service providers seeing themselves as experts, little room is allowed for clients to shape and direct intervention using the rehabilitation model. The client may be seen as the focus of attention; however, she is often afforded little control of what happens. Performance deficits identified by the professional define the nature of interventions provided.[22] In the rehabilitation model, the priority for treatment is restoration of function except in cases where it is obvious that function cannot be regained, such as with the loss of a limb. Education is provided to increase compliance with treatment,[22] the assumption being that once people understand *why* things are being done, they will automatically agree to do it.

The role of technology for restoring body structure and function and remediation frequently captures the attention of funding bodies and rehabilitation professionals. After all, this provides the potential for the problem being remediated "permanently." Unfortunately, whereas this high-end technology is being developed and funded, the role of technology to enable people in everyday life is often overshadowed. Assistive technologies, frequently presented as the final intervention in the hierarchy of treatment, are perceived as the last resort and frequently left to discharge planning. When technology is prescribed, it is in response to the specific deficits present,[20] that is, whatever the person is able or not able to do, rather than in terms of what he or she *wants* to do or the context in which activities are to be performed. Until recently, wheelchairs have been primarily designed to replace walking, not to enable people to mobilize in a variety of environments such as through the bush or along a beach. The rehabilitation model does not easily accommodate the unique goals and interests of the person, the nature of the activities in which they wish to engage, or the environments in which the technology is to be used.

Outcomes in the rehabilitation model are defined and evaluated by service providers[22] and are usually focused on achieving an ideal performance standard or complete independence. Measuring the success of a technology outcome is difficult in this model, as many of the standardized tests for independence consider independence to be compromised with the use of technology. For example, the highest score of 7 can only be achieved on the Functional Independence Measure (FIM)[52] by people who do not require any assistance or use a device to complete the task.[11] In addition, evaluating the quality of the outcome of independence is not possible, as the FIM is a global construct that merely requires the task to be completed without assistance. Little attention is given to the quality or acceptability of the performance. For example, some people with disabilities believe the time and effort required to complete self-care activities would be better spent on other more personally rewarding tasks.

Abandonment and nonuse of AT devices are major concerns.[4,20,28,29,35,43] Follow-up studies consistently report that 30% to 50% of assistive devices recommended, such as hearing aids and mobility and self-care equipment, are abandoned.[44] Factors observed to influence continued use of a device include consumer involvement in device selection; change in the priorities or needs of the user; motivation to use the device or do the task; environmental obstacles; and whether the device was seen as effective, reliable, durable, comfortable, and easy to use.[13,19,27,36,41,44,47] Psychosocial factors, such as the social acceptability of the device and the degree to which the device heightens the visibility of disability, also have been proposed as key factors in the acceptance of assistive technologies.[8,20]

Technology abandonment has serious repercussions. After abandoning AT devices, people with disabilities may perform less than optimally, and scarce resources have been wasted. As service providers, we lay the responsibility for abandonment on the user rather than examining our roles in making an inappropriate match.[14] A better understanding of the process of choosing, matching, and using AT devices,[37,44] as well as a closer examination of services involved in the process,[17] is necessary to improve service delivery.

■ NEEDS-BASED APPROACH TO TECHNOLOGY APPLICATION

In response to the problems previously noted in the use of AT devices, AT professionals sought to augment the rehabilitation model with one that addressed issues related to selecting technology. In addition, antidiscrimination legislation and return-to-work policies and programs, which assisted people with disabilities in returning to mainstream employment, moved AT services to a new context—the community. Models that worked well in medical environments did not translate well into these new service environments. Service providers also grappled with an explosion of new devices, a complex matrix of services, and the inadequacies of the rehabilitation model to deal with the pragmatics of identifying and selecting an assistive technology solution in the real world. This led a number of experienced clinicians to develop models to guide people through the process of technology acquisition.[2,31,49] These procedures, in combination with individualized rehabilitation or educational plans, unified the diverse assistive technology services and providers by outlining a systematic process and detailing the steps involved in selecting technology. In these models, service providers are encouraged to be aware of the whole AT process and to ensure that the user is informed throughout the entire process and has access to appropriate support at each stage. The progression is presented as linear and involves many steps (Box 2-1).

As proposed, the order of these steps may vary and each may not be required in all situations.[49] Although primarily procedural, needs-based models

---

BOX 2-1

Steps to the Assistive Technology Process

1. Identify the tasks
2. Identify the consumer's abilities
3. Identify possible assistive technology devices (ATDs)
4. Identify present and future environments
5. Evaluate the interface between the consumer and ATD
6. Select the ATD by all team members
7. Train the consumer to use and maintain the ATD
8. Document the evaluation process
9. Periodically reevaluate all parts of the AT system

From Bain BK, Leger D: *Assistive Technology: An Interdisciplinary Approach.* New York, Churchill Livingstone, 1997.

---

detail elements and hold underlying assumptions that affect service delivery that bear closer examination. Needs-based models propose that people have individual goals and seek to engage in everyday activities. An individual's needs are defined by identifying activities he or she wishes to perform within a specific environment, and by developing a good definition of functional goals or needs.[49] Some needs-based models also highlight barriers in the environment (e.g., auditing the physical environment for accessibility)[2,50] and address elements in the environment likely to impinge on an activity or intervention.[2] These models encourage users to be involved through use of interviews to assist them in specifying their needs.[32,49] However, clinicians also analyze the essential elements of the job and use physical and functional ability measures to assess capacity to fulfill task performance requirements.[2,49,50] Observation also is an important source of information, allowing clinicians to evaluate the consumer's actual task performance.[2] These models primarily focus on the individual's presenting needs and use a problem-solving approach to improve function. The goal of intervention is to enhance a person's ability, comfort, and function.[49] Service providers are involved, as appropriate, with one clinician taking the responsibility for coordinating or managing the "case."

A range of interventions are used with simple, cost-effective solutions taking priority. Symms and Ross outlined a hierarchy of assistive technology[51] and advised that the preferred hierarchy for interventions should be less costly items, such as modifying or revising a job, followed by (1) creative utilization of commercial devices, (2) use of commercially available rehabilitation products, then (3) combining technologies, (4) modifying existing commercial options, and finally (5) fabricating new devices. If a device is required, the abilities, needs, and desires of the user are matched with the device features and available funding to identify the best option. The expected outcome of a needs-based model would be that the needs identified by the consumer are met. The success of the outcomes would be determined by the AT user's level of satisfaction with the device. In some cases, the user's level of satisfaction with the AT device and overall process would also be sought to determine adequacy of the services delivered.

Working with Steven Using a Needs-Based Model

In light of the previous description of needs-based models, the implications of using this model in addressing Steven's technology needs can be addressed by asking the following questions:
- How would a service provider using a rehabilitation framework view Steven?
- How would his needs be defined?
- What assessment processes would Steven experience?
- What interventions or services would be available to him?
- How would the service provider relate to Steven?
- How would the technology be selected and applied?

Needs-based models provide a practical approach to meeting Steven's technology needs. In this model, Steven and the service providers are aware of the steps involved in selecting the technology. Despite the diversity of their expertise, the service providers possess a common vision of the sequence of events and their contribution to the process. Steven would work with a primary practitioner to identify and engage other service providers, as appropriate. In this model, Steven is seen as having individual priorities and goals. Therefore, service providers would seek his input to develop intervention goals and be interested in his understanding of the job and task requirements if he had been working in the same position prior to his injury. If Steven did not have prior experience of the position, the service provider would undertake a job analysis and assess Steven's capacity to fulfill essential elements of the job. Steven's capacities may be addressed with use of standardized work performance tests and/or observation in situ. The service provider would then problem-solve the presenting issues and seek to enhance Steven's ability, comfort, and function in the workplace. A range of interventions may be suggested, such as reassigning tasks, alternative strategies, new mainstream technologies, assistive devices, training, using support personnel, and redesigning or modifying the environment. Device requirements are likely to be determined by Steven's abilities and preferences, the funding available, and aspects of the environment, which impact on his return to work (e.g., accessibility of the building, use of technology, compatibility with existing computer platforms). Steven, and possibly his employer, would then be asked to indicate his level of satisfaction with the interventions and the process. His satisfaction would be revisited at a later stage to check if the interventions are still working well for him. Table 2-2 identifies Steven's needs and technology requirements within the needs-based model.

Implications of a Needs-Based Model for Assistive Technology Users

As an example of procedural models, the needs-based model provides a systematic framework for an often overwhelming process. In detailing the process, the model enables AT users and service providers to understand the steps required

TABLE 2-2

Defining Steven's AT Requirements Using the Needs-Based Model

DEFINED NEEDS	TECHNOLOGY REQUIREMENTS/CHARACTERISTICS
Access to computer	Hand/finger splints, trackerball Modified desk
Mobilize around the school, classrooms, and playing fields	Wheelchair with good maneuverability
Well-supported seated position all day	Roho cushion
Access to relevant facilities in the school	Ramp to staff room Accessible toilet in staff area

to identify and select an appropriate technology. This practical approach has the potential to offer AT users opportunities to express their needs; however, the level of control they have over the process is contingent on many factors. First, the level of collaboration between the user and the clinician will frequently depend on the control the clinician affords them. In needs-based models, AT users are perceived as having individual goals and needs and should therefore set the goals and direct the process. However, while the clinician might espouse being client-centered, the manner in which assessment and intervention strategies are undertaken may not afford the client control. For example, when undertaking complex tests to define performance requirements the service provider may use these results to override the AT user's perception of the job's requirements or their abilities. In addition, the diverse range of equipment and pressure on the service to identify a cost-effective solution quickly may mean that the service provider selects a minimal set of devices for the user to choose from.

Second, control is usually in the hands of the person with knowledge. For many novice users and clinicians alike, having a full appreciation of the extensive range of options available is difficult. Consequently, an inexperienced user would be dependent on the AT practitioner to provide sufficient knowledge to contribute to decisions. Similarly an inexperienced practitioner may deflect responsibility for identifying suitable options onto the user (regardless of their expertise).

Third, experience and problem-solving capacity determine what and how issues are addressed. Without experience, appreciating the complex matrix of factors affecting performance is difficult, if not impossible. Textbook solutions do not always resolve or apply to idiosyncratic real-world issues. Therapists and AT users frequently rely on trial and error, their natural aptitude for problem solving, or information and strategies accumulated from years of experience to deal with problems. The center of control rests with the person who has the best understanding of the issues and skills in developing practical solutions.

Finally, funding also determines how the AT user's technology needs are met. The capacity of the service provider to respond to the user's needs also depends on the context in which the service is being provided and the resources available. For example, because of the way in which funding is made available, AT users can access service providers and funding to address their technology needs at work or for further education, but would have to self-fund services and equipment for leisure activities. In addition, the funding available and the goals of the funder and service provider determine the quality of the solution. Priorities for simplicity and cost effectiveness can overshadow user preferences and the quality of performance required by the AT user in the workplace.

Needs-based models, with their focus on process, concentrate on immediate issues, as few conceptual models deal with the often overwhelming complexities in identifying the long-term technology requirements of an employee with a disability. This lack of conceptualization means no frameworks are available to describe factors affecting the AT user or assess the quality of the intervention.

In needs-based models, technology is one of a range of options explored, and selection of the best technology is dependent on an understanding of the AT user's requirements and preferences, having extensive knowledge of the assistive devices available, their features, and performance trade-offs.[49] Although needs-based models have provided useful frameworks for identifying and selecting technology, they do not provide a structure for implementing technology, which is integrating the technology into the application environment and addressing ongoing issues that are inevitable. Aspects of the environment that affect the user's return to work, such as accessibility of the building and use of technology, also would need to be addressed. However, issues related to integration of the AT user into the workplace, understanding the expectations of the employer and coworkers, and mechanisms for dealing with future changes would remain unattended unless the service provider had extensive experience. One advantage of these needs-based models is that they do stipulate that the effectiveness of the technology must be evaluated. Thus, outcomes are measured in terms of how well the intervention meets the goals of the user. This underscores the importance of clearly and thoroughly defining the needs of the users up front. In addition, user satisfaction with the technology and process are evaluated but generally only at the time the solution is put in place.

NEED FOR SOUND THEORETICAL FOUNDATION IN ASSISTIVE TECHNOLOGY

Although the needs-based model reflects the intention of AT service providers to refine service delivery and develop guidelines for identifying appropriate technology, competent practice requires a sound theoretical foundation.[21] Theories help to translate the intuitive experience of practitioners into testable, systematically organized concepts and variables. Theories describe and explain phenomena and how they are related. Theories form the foundation of conceptual models, which provide a structure for current knowledge, as well as examining and integrating new parameters.[25] Conceptual models, based on theories, then provide a means of maintaining quality by providing a structure for planning and evaluating interventions and services.[25] AT practice requires conceptual models to describe the broad range of elements involved in the selection and integration of AT and how they interact to ensure that the technology solution continues to work well in the context.

Any conceptual system developed for AT services should complement the values of society and the culture in which we work. Further, these models must operate within the relevant service systems.[34] Models should ensure the practitioner is providing relevant services, consistent with consumer expectations and legislative requirements.[39] In recent years, two major movements have affected AT service delivery. First, the International Classification of Functioning, Disability and Health (ICF) has resulted in a new conceptualization and definition of disability.[56] Second, a change in the expectations of consumers has resulted from the independent living movement and consumerism. Contemporary AT models need to reflect these changes so that relevant AT services are provided to consumers in a way that is acceptable to them.

Traditionally, the individual model of disability was the predominant way of thinking about impairment and disability. As noted in the rehabilitation model, disablement was viewed as a personal problem, directly caused by disease, trauma, or health conditions, that required medical care provided by professionals in the form of individual treatment.[57] More recently, the ICF has promoted an alternative model of disability requiring a philosophical shift in the way disability is perceived and how people with disabilities are treated.[56] First, the ICF focuses on health states rather than personal deficits. Seen as more than an absence of disease, health is regarded as being satisfied with life and having a sense of well-being.[22] Second, the ICF recognizes that people vary enormously in background, coping styles, habits, and lifestyle, thereby acknowledging that people have diverse needs that require varying responses or solutions. Third, in defining health, the ICF requires that we move beyond attending to the impaired body structures and function to enabling people to engage in activities and participate fully in society. Fourth, and most importantly, disability is not viewed as an attribute of the person, but rather as a consequence of the environment.

This social model of disability locates the problem of disability and the responsibility for dealing with it within society. Disability is not seen as the result of limitations of an individual,[33] but rather as the inability of society to accommodate the diversity of abilities in the community. The social model has redefined disability in terms of disabling environments and promoted people with a disability as citizens with rights.[16]

The philosophical shift precipitated by the ICF requires that AT models be founded on an understanding of well-being rather than impairment and deficits. The ICF requires AT models to account for the unique experiences, goals, and interests of each person and investigate the role of technology in enabling people to do what they *want* to do and participate equitably in society. Further, it challenges AT service providers to understand the barriers that exist in the environment and to take responsibility for removing barriers to technology use and participation in the community.

In parallel with the development of the ICF, consumers have sought more control over the nature of services available and the way in which they are offered. Antidiscrimination, equal opportunity, and disability services legislation has resulted in consumers demanding control, personal choice, and inclusion at all levels of service delivery.[9] This shift in philosophy has called for a change in professional-consumer relationships and models of service delivery[5,7] with a focus on client-centered practice. Three basic assumptions that underpin a client-centered approach are: (1) clients and their families are unique, (2) they know themselves best, and (3) optimal function is most likely in a supportive family and community context.[5]

Client-centered services require that clients determine the goals and outcomes of interventions and define their priorities together with service providers.[21] Service models must therefore enable clients to participate equitably in the process, have control over the outcome,[18] and use their natural community supports.[5] Although some authors have advocated that clients should drive decision making and be empowered to achieve solutions for themselves, others have proposed that some clients require a more structured form of client-centered interventions.[21] For example, service providers may need to facilitate consumer involvement and decision making.[5] AT models must provide a framework for services that will (1) ensure interventions are founded on the user's goals, (2) enable users to understand factors that affect the success of an AT intervention, (3) empower users to guide or direct the AT process to achieve their preferred outcome, and (4) allow existing supports in the community to be identified and effectively utilized.

It is apparent, after examining the models of service delivery proposed to date, that the deficit-centered paradigms, such as rehabilitation models, predominate. These models continue to focus on the limitations of the individual rather than examining environmental variables that contribute to their disability.[9] With the focus being on the individual, little attention has been paid to the interplay of multiple factors that affect the AT system and contribute to the potential success or failure of the system. Though recognized as central to this system, the AT user is not able to be an active part of the decision making if he or she is perceived as the recipient of services or as having deficits that need to be defined and measured.

Recently, a number of contemporary AT models have been developed that focus on how technology can be used to enable people to participate equitably in society. These models provide a broader understanding of factors that affect technology use. Rather than seeing technology as a means of accommodating lost function, they examine how technology can assist people to participate in activities and environments. They also provide AT practitioners and consumers with a framework for systematically addressing barriers to technology use frequently encountered in the selection and application of technology.

▇ HOLISTIC APPROACH TO TECHNOLOGY APPLICATION

In line with the ICF, the Human Activities and Assistive Technology (HAAT) Model[11] focuses on enabling people to accomplish what they want to do by examining the activities in which they wish to participate and the environments in which these activities occur. The HAAT model is concerned with using technology to enable *someone* (a person with a disability) to do *something* (an activity) *somewhere* (in the environment).[11] The HAAT model draws on a generic human performance model proposed initially by Bailey,[1] which was developed "to assist in the design and application of technology" (p. 37).[11] In an attempt to explain the interplay of factors in technology design and use, Cook and Hussey adapted Bailey's model to explain the interrelationship between the activity, the AT user, the AT, and the environment (Figure 2-1). They referred to the interplay of these elements as the Assistive Technology (AT) System. The activity defines the goal of the system, which, in combination with the environment, defines the requirements for task completion. AT is seen as a means of enabling the person with different capacities to complete a task in a particular context. AT, although adapted to the person's requirements, the task, and the environment, also places demands on the system that need to be addressed. Cook and Hussey[11] emphasize the importance of the interplay between these factors throughout the whole process of acquiring and integrating the AT. The AT system is seen as an open system, which is dynamic and interacts with the environment. Over time, changes may occur in the activity, person, technology, or context that will alter the way functions are allocated within the system. For example, the person may develop additional skills or lose abilities, requiring the use of different or additional technologies. Alternatively, a change in the activity or environment may place additional demands on the system. Further, advances

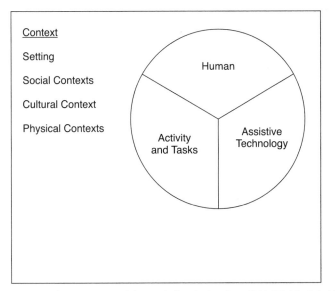

FIGURE 2-1 ■ The Human Activity Assistive Technology (HAAT) Model. (Adapted from Cook AM, Hussey SM: *Assistive Technologies: Principles and Practice,* ed 2. St. Louis, Mosby, 2002.)

in technology may mean that more sophisticated functions are available to the user, or that incompatibilities arise as the workplace platform is upgraded.

By identifying the elements in the AT system, the HAAT model holds the AT practitioner responsible for achieving the user's goals and establishing a *good fit* between the activities, user, technology, and environment. The AT practitioner is guided to examine the user's life roles and tasks involved in his/her daily work, leisure, and self-care activities. Each user is seen as a unique person with biological structures that enable him to sense, process, and act, as well as having skills, abilities, and experiences that he brings to the system. The AT user is seen as the operator and, therefore, in charge of the AT system. Issues and problems arise as a result of the inability of a person to participate in his preferred or required activities. The model encourages service providers to examine the interface between the AT and the user; activities; and the physical, social, and cultural environment to ensure a good fit. The role of the service provider is to provide consumers and their teams with sufficient information to make informed choices. The service provider brings specialist knowledge and expertise to collaborations with users and other stakeholders involved in the process.

In the assessment process, information is gathered about the skills and abilities of the user, activities to be performed, and the contexts in which they are undertaken, and then the user's ability to use the mutually selected assistive technology. Assessment is seen as an ongoing process rather than a discrete event. Progress toward goals is continuously reevaluated using reflection-in-action to continuously revise interventions as difficulties or new information arises. Cook and Hussey advocate that assessments focus on the strengths and abilities of the user.[11] Qualitative and quantitative measures are used in the form of interviews, functional evaluations, observations, and criterion-referenced performance measures.

The goal of intervention is to enable the person to achieve her goal. However, Cook and Hussey do acknowledge the value of using parallel interventions to improve the individual's skill level as well as to enable function.[11] Interventions can include low- and high-tech options and hard or soft technologies. Technologies are not seen as a means of rehabilitating or remediating impairment, but rather as enabling the person to perform the functional activities she desires to perform. Alternative strategies or personal assistance can also be used to meet specific needs, according to Cook and Hussey.[11] Although some propose assistive technology should be considered before personal assistance,[53] Cook and Hussey recommend that the preferred choice of the individual be used.[11] Intervention should be aimed at both meeting the user's current needs and seeking to predict the user's future technology needs.

Successful completion of the functional activity in the application environment demonstrates the success of the AT system. The effectiveness of the AT system is determined by measuring the performance of the system, that is, the ability of the person to complete the activity successfully using the assistive technology in the application environment.[11] The person's satisfaction with the intervention and the process also are important outcome considerations. In addition, the impact of the AT system on the person's quality of life is considered.

Working with Steven Using the HAAT Model

In light of the previous description of the HAAT model, we now return to consider the implications of using this model in addressing Steven's technology needs. Some questions that arise include the following:

- How would a service provider using a rehabilitation framework view him?
- How would a service provider define Steven's needs?
- What assessment processes would Steven experience?
- What interventions or services would be available to Steven?
- How would the service provider relate to him?
- How would the technology be selected and applied in this context?

When using the HAAT model, Steven's technology needs would be identified with reference to his unique goals, skills, abilities, and experience. The service provider would explore Steven's satisfaction with his performance in daily activities and focus on activities he prioritizes, working with him and his team to identify potential solutions. A good understanding of the physical, social, and cultural aspects of the application environment or environments would be sought to identify potential demands on the system and to ensure the technology can be adequately supported. Steven would be interviewed and his abilities related to technology use assessed through formal or criterion-referenced performance measures, as well as real-world observation. Steven would be provided with information on a range of options, including high- and low-tech devices, hard and soft technologies, and the value of alternative strategies and personal assistance would also be discussed with him.

Steven's performance using various solutions would be observed and evaluated to discuss the strengths and limitation of each solution to meet his requirements. Throughout the process, the interaction between Steven, his activities, the AT, and his environment would be continuously reevaluated to ensure a good fit is achieved. Steven would gain a good sense of his capabilities and the potential of technology to enable him to achieve his goals. He would be provided with opportunities to further develop his skills and potential to use the technology. Discussions would explore his future goals and anticipated changes in technology in the upcoming years. The service provider also would explore with Steven how the technology under consideration could be used to empower him in other aspects of his life and application environments. The final solution would be decided in consultation with Steven, after discussing how well it fits with Steven's skills, abilities, and experience, the range of activities with which it will be used, other technologies with which it is likely to interface, and how well it fits with the physical, social, and cultural aspects of the application environment. Through this experience, the service provider would aim to make Steven aware of the factors that have an impact on the technology and empower him to deal with these as issues arise. However, provision would be made to follow up with Steven to address his changing needs and update his solutions as other technologies become available. The success of the intervention would be determined by how well Steven is able to perform the activities in the application environment immediately after purchase, as well as long term. Steven's and the employer's satisfaction with the technology and the process would also be examined. Table 2-3 identifies Steven's needs and technology requirements within the HAAT model.

Impact of the HAAT Model on Assistive Technology Users

The concepts in the HAAT model translate well into clinical practice. They provide AT practitioners with a structure for systematically addressing factors that affect the AT system and exploring the factors likely to affect the success or failure of an AT intervention. This model allows issues to be identified in relation to the individual's skills, abilities, and experiences, the activities and tasks of the job, the AT, and the physical, sociocultural, and personal-social aspects of the

TABLE 2-3
Defining Steven's AT Requirements Using the HAAT Model

DEFINED NEEDS	TECHNOLOGY REQUIREMENTS/CHARACTERISTICS
PERSON	
PE teacher — active person	Transportable
Husband and father to two children (6 and 8 years)	Multiple users
Enjoys playing games on Playstation	Games capacity
Low-tech literacy/experience; interested in developing skills	User friendly with room to accommodate skill development
Difficulty using standard keyboard/mouse	Hand/finger splints, trackball voice recognition
Stable posture but some tenderness in buttock at end of day	Roho cushion
ACTIVITY	
Word processing (speed requirement "to type as fast as he can think")	Speed enhancement
Internet access likely in the near future	Efficient mouse alternative
Mobilizes around the school, classrooms, and grounds	Wheelchair with good maneuverability Accessible paths of travel and doorways
TECHNOLOGY	
Network system	Technologies need to be compatible with network and ensure acceptable level of security to system
ENVIRONMENT	
School largely ground level but playing fields rough	Wheelchair tires that can handle outside terrain
Shares office space with other teachers	Multiple users
Access to relevant facilities in the school	Accessible paths of travel and adequate circulation spaces, accessible toilet

environment, as well as the interaction between these elements. Having developed from a generic model of human performance using computer technology,[1] conceptually the model does not encourage a clinical perspective or a focus on deficits. In line with the ICF definition of disability, this model encourages practitioners to focus on enabling participation and defining performance as a mismatch between the user, AT, and the environment, rather than being defined as a human impairment or deficit. This model allows the unique aspects of the users and their contexts to be considered by identifying individual goals and implementing tailored technology solutions. Furthermore, since the functioning of the AT system is the primary focus of this model, ongoing revision of its effectiveness can be integrated into service delivery. Interestingly, Cook and Hussey favor an "educational model" for service delivery, although they do encourage "client-driven" outcome measurement. They propose that this model should move away from the traditional "expert model," assuming that the consumer relies on the service provider to supply information and guidance through the process. Although some users would certainly appreciate this support, more experienced consumers may find the paternalism of this approach restrictive.

Cook and Hussey provide a detailed description of the model in their text *Assistive Technology: Principles and Practice*. They outline a range of assessment tools and protocols to assist service providers in operationalizing the model.[11] Being a primarily human factors model, the strength of this model is in analyzing and operationalizing technology solutions. Consequently, Cook and Hussey provide a detailed description of how to assess the human-technology interface and understand the features and demands of the technology. In doing this, the HAAT model strongly emphasizes the mechanics of the AT system and focuses less on the personal and environmental aspects of the model. The authors do, however, discuss the application of technology in the educational and vocational context and outline procedural and environmental considerations in these settings. The HAAT model provides AT service providers with an intuitive and holistic approach to addressing people's technology needs.[25] The detailed description of AT assists practitioners in selecting and applying technologies and understanding the demands these devices place on the user, to better prepare the user to apply technology effectively. With a deep understanding of the power and potential of technology, users and service providers are better prepared to anticipate future needs. The user is empowered to effectively apply the technology in all aspects of his life. Although the HAAT model specifically identifies AT as an explicit component in the model,[24] it would work equally well for any strategy designed to enable the user, such as alternative strategies or personal assistance. Use of the HAAT model would permit an evaluation of how these alternative strategies interface with the person, activities, and environment. This would require that the AT section of the pie be replaced with an assistive mechanism or system.

Unfortunately, the HAAT model is descriptive rather than predictive. Although the authors contend that systematic consideration of all four elements will ensure success of the AT system,[24] this conceptual model has not been tested to date. In addition, within the HAAT model, no assessment or outcomes measures have been developed, which would enable the performance of the system to be evaluated. Cook and Hussey, however, refer practitioners to other models and tools (e.g., Matching Person and Technology [MPT] model[43]) and assessment instruments such as the Canadian Occupational Performance Measure (COPM)[23] as appropriate to address various elements in the model. They also identify validated measures developed specifically for evaluating AT outcomes, such as the Quebec User Evaluation of Satisfaction with Assistive Technology (QUEST)[15] and Psychosocial Impact of Assistive Devices Scale (PIADS).[14]

▓ USERS' PERSONAL PERSPECTIVES TOWARD ASSISTIVE TECHNOLOGY

In the last few years, people with disabilities have begun to reflect on their experiences with AT and redirect service providers' attention from merely selecting technology to the issues they experience *using* it. Although service providers are focused on the value of AT in improving function, improved function does not by itself ensure AT use.[13,35,41] Cushman and Scherer found consumers to be less positive about the aesthetic aspects of devices than the service providers, although they appreciated their functional benefits.[13] While the perceived usefulness or aesthetics of the device influence whether it is accepted or rejected, many consumers fear the stigma attached to using a device that visibly defines them as being different or as having an identifiable disability.[7,12] An overly negative or positive perception of AT affects the person's self-perception and value of the device.[8] The outcome of varying consumer views is that some people with disabilities decline to use AT despite its many advantages.[12] For example, even though he had vision impairment all his life, Covington only started using a white cane in adulthood. It took a month using the cane for him to feel more independent and learn to accept the aid rather than regarding it as a barrier. Personal sources of meaning attributed to devices such as the person's history of and experience with support use, the meaning of specific activities, and the cultural meaning associated with particular tools also have been identified as affecting people's willingness to acquire and use AT.[48] Limited research exists on AT users' perspectives, and the studies that do exist are largely descriptive and scattered throughout a variety of sources. This literature does, however, reflect a diversity of experience.[7] A greater appreciation of the user's perspective is required if we are to understand AT users and empower them to choose the technology that addresses their needs, preferences, and their ongoing concerns, at the same time recognizing the role of the environment in disabling or enabling them.

▓ UNDERSTANDING TECHNOLOGY USE

AT users are as different and diverse as anyone else in the community. Even when using similar technologies, people differ in the way in which they use them and the purposes for which they use them. Some people have a great inclination for using technology and others have no interest in it. Furthermore, people may avoid using technologies in one context while embracing them in another. No universal formula exists for selecting technology; however, the active participation of the user is critical to the success of the technology in achieving the individual's goals.[6] Getting to know the AT user and his or her capabilities and concerns has been identified as critical to a client-centered approach to identifying the best AT system for an individual.[6,43] Although the HAAT model provides a framework for addressing the interface between the technology, activity, user, and environment, and how these affect the AT system, it does not yet provide a deep understanding of how the interaction between the user, technology, and the environment affects technology use.

▨ MATCHING PERSON AND TECHNOLOGY MODEL

One model that attempts to explain the psychosocial aspects of technology use is the MPT Model.[43] This model grew out of grounded-theory research that examined use and nonuse of AT by adults with physical disabilities.[25] The MPT model presents three layers of factors that impact AT use. In the first level are the environment, characteristics of the person, and features of the device. The next level consists of expectations and definitions of rehabilitation success by and for that individual, the person's view of his or her present and future quality of life, and his or her experience of disability. The outer layer of this model reflects the interaction among the physiologic, psychological and psychosocial determinants of disability (Figure 2-2).

The MPT model highlights the importance of understanding the person, technology, and milieu to make a good match. It provides a range of tools to examine each of these factors in detail. This model focuses the AT practitioner on the user's personality, temperament, and preferences; the salient characteristics of the technology; the expectations, support, and opportunities afforded by the environment or milieu; and how these impact potential technology use. The MPT model acknowledges that people with disabilities cope with illness and impairments in a variety of ways, and that different strategies are required to assist them in adjusting and coping with difficulties and change. It examines the personal aspects of the AT user, that is, his or her experience with, attitude toward, and capacity to use technology, and seeks to identify characteristics in the technology that best match these.

Problems are defined in the MPT model in terms of the potential nonuse of technology. Although Scherer does not promote MPT as a predictive model,[25] this model directs service providers to examine factors associated with use and nonuse drawn from the author's consumer-focused research. Scherer's model is designed to ensure that the process of technology selection is user driven and person centered. The constructs and assessment tools in this model provide a foundation for consumers to explore their perceptions of AT. The service provider is seen as a collaborator who assists the AT user to understand the factors most likely to influence his or her technology use. This model provides a structure for the user's goals and preferences to be considered in the process of device selection. It encourages consumers to be involved early in the process of device evaluation and selection by having them fill in self-report checklists,

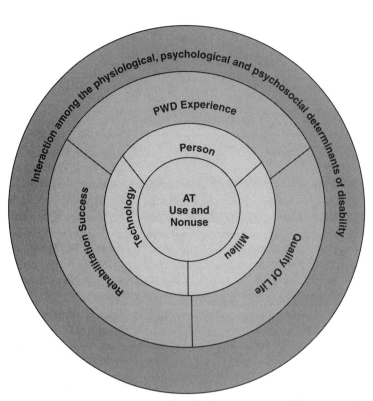

FIGURE 2-2 ■ The Matching Person and Technology (MPT) model. (From Scherer MJ: The impact of assistive technology on the lives of people with disabilities, in Gray DB, Quatrano LA, Lieberman ML (eds): *Designing and Using Assistive Technology: The Human Perspective.* Baltimore, Paul H. Brookes, 1998.)

which examine their perceptions of technology and predisposition to technology use. These checklists then provide a blueprint for ensuring that the technology is "a realistic and appealing match for that particular user" (p. 130).[45] This model examines whether specific goals are achieved without pain, fatigue, or stress. The service provider also uses an instrument to assess the technology needs of the user and the degree to which the user's and provider's perspectives match and are openly considered in the selection of a device.

MPT allows the user and service provider to consider very carefully whether technology is an appropriate solution for the person in her current context. If technology is considered to be appropriate, the model provides a structure for examining and comparing options and determining acceptable tradeoffs. Technology is viewed as providing potential advantages and disadvantages to the user. Technology is considered in terms of its design; that is, its usability, compatibility, cost-effectiveness, reliability, and appeal, as well as the accompanying service supports. Aspects of the application environment also are a focus of the intervention, which is attending to the physical and attitudinal issues that will affect technology use. Outcome measures in this model examine use and nonuse, user satisfaction, and user's perceived well-being.[25]

Working with Steven Using the MPT Model

In light of the previous description of the MPT model, we now return to consider the implications of using this model in addressing Steven's technology needs. Some questions that arise include:

- How would a service provider using a rehabilitation framework view Steven?
- How would a service provider define his needs?
- What assessment processes would Steven experience?
- What interventions or services would be available to him?
- How would the service provider relate to Steven?
- How would the technology be selected and applied?

Using the MPT model the service provider would be interested in understanding Steven's general coping strategies as well as his experience with, attitude toward, and capacity to use technology. In addition, information would be sought on the physical and attitudinal aspects of the environment related to technology use. Steven would complete a series of questionnaires, which would prompt him to consider and comment on his current and future goals and use of technology. The service provider would then work with Steven to examine the potential value to him of technology use. Steven would be guided through a process to identify the key characteristic of technology best suited to his goals, preferences, and milieu, and be provided with checklists to assist him in considering his technology options. Steven would be alerted to factors most likely to have an impact on his technology use and collaborate with the service provider to address these in his choice of technology or in developing the necessary supports. The effectiveness of the intervention is evaluated in terms of Steven's perception of the adequacy of the process, satisfaction with the device, and, ultimately, use or nonuse of the technology. Table 2-4 identifies Steven's needs and technology requirements within the MPT model.

Impact of the MPT Model on AT Users

The MPT model uses a "whole of life" approach, which acknowledges individual differences and encourages users to examine the place of technology in their lives. This model provides a structure that allows the AT user to be involved in the process of device selection from the very outset and assists her to examine her abilities, level of satisfaction with her current technology use, and whether a device is potentially useful. When determining appropriate technology, the model focuses on the user, her function and attitude to technology, and the social milieu of the person's environment and its role in impeding or facilitating the use of technology. This model is largely interested in assessing the interaction between the technology, user, and the physical and attitudinal environment as related to defined goals. Although it enables the user to examine the application of technology across her life and in various application environments, it does not provide a structure for examining the specific requirements of each activity

TABLE 2-4

Defining Steven's AT Requirements Using the MPT Model

DEFINED NEEDS	TECHNOLOGY REQUIREMENTS/CHARACTERISTICS
USER	
PE teacher — active person	Transportable
Husband and father to two children (6 and 8 years)	Multiple users
Positive mood and outlook, preferences and priorities, all compatible with technology use and successful performance	Complex technology may be tolerated
Enjoys playing games on Playstation	Games capacity
Low-tech literacy/experience; interested in developing skills	User friendly with room to accommodate skill development
Difficulty using standard keyboard/mouse	Alternative means of computer input and navigation
Stable posture but some tenderness in buttock at end of day	Pressure management system for seat
TECHNOLOGY	
Network system	Technologies need to be compatible with network and ensure acceptable level of security to system
ENVIRONMENT	
School largely ground level but playing fields rough	Wheelchair tires that can handle outside terrain
Shares office space with other teachers	Multiple users
Access to relevant facilities in the school	Accessible paths of travel and adequate circulation spaces, accessible toilets
Support from others available	Complex system may be supported

(e.g., how the technologies required for Internet access may differ from word processing). Furthermore, because it is focused on examining the value of technology, the model itself does not provide a facility for examining the value of alternative solutions to the presenting issue (e.g., alternative strategies, reassigning tasks, or personal assistance).

The assessment instruments developed by Scherer have been very useful to service providers and are the first validated tools to address the person, technology, and environmental fit. Vincent and Morin concluded that items from the *Assistive Technology Device Predisposition Assessment (ATD PA)* "focus well on the pertinent factors related to individuals' decisions to use or not use an assistive technology" (p. 100).[54] MPT assessments also have been used to compare users' attitudes to and expectations of AT with subsequent use.[13] Additionally the assessment tools are useful for identifying users' experiences and perceptions of AT and to compare them with those of service providers,[13] especially the differences in their perceived value of devices. The ability of these tools to predict technology abandonment has great potential, but has only recently been empirically demonstrated.[43b] However, the model does provide the structure for examining outcomes across multiple activities.

The capacity of the MPT model to address the concerns of the AT user lies in the way in which it is applied. If embedded in an impairment model of disability, the service provider's focus would be on the person's reaction to disability or his or her temperament, which would then be seen as hindering the acceptance of AT. If the assessment tools are not used correctly, the service provider may be tempted to make value judgments about users and their attitudes toward the technology, defining people's attitudes toward technology in terms of their predisposition. This suggests a way of determining someone's suitability for technology and potential for success or failure. In reality, a person's attitude toward technology may vary, depending on the nature of the activity being undertaken, the capacity of the technology to perform various functions effectively, and how well it is supported in any given context. A practitioner who works from a social model of disability and embraces client-centered practice is well placed to use the MPT model's user-driven approach and accompanying tools to empower the AT user to decide if technology is an appropriate solution and to understand the personal and environmental factors that require consideration when choosing the technology.

MAINSTREAM MODELS OF TECHNOLOGY APPLICATION

Research on mainstream technologies could contribute a great deal to AT practice.[38] For many years businesses have tried to facilitate effective technology use. Technology has become a routine part of everyday life, so knowing how to help people accept technologies and use them effectively is vital. In addition, mainstream technologies are developing capabilities proving to be invaluable to people with disabilities. The question is no longer focused solely on whether technology is suitable and what technologies are available to meet the user's goals. We are now seeking to understand which of the many options available provide the user with the most efficient and versatile solution and how the user can be further enabled to make the best use of the technology. A wealth of research has been undertaken to inform the development and application of mainstream technologies. Two approaches have the potential to contribute to AT service delivery, namely, human-centered design and attributional theory.

Human-centered design focuses on the usability of technology and is recognized as being crucial to the success of technology.[26] Similar to the HAAT model, this approach is interested in developing a technology system or device that meets the needs of the user, the tasks to be undertaken, as well as the environment, including its technical, physical, and organizational elements. The approach requires designers to analyze the context of technology use to design a usable solution. Design models have moved from being primarily focused on meeting task requirements to those that consider the technical and physical environment, understanding the user, and the organization context. The main elements of a context analysis proposed by Maguire are outlined in Box 2-2.

BOX 2-2
Context of Use Factors

User Group
- System skills and experience
- Task knowledge
- Training
- Qualifications
- Language skills
- Age and gender
- Physical and cognitive capabilities
- Attitudes and motivations

Tasks
- Task list
- Goal
- Output
- Steps
- Frequency
- Importance
- Duration
- Dependencies

Technical Environment
- Auditory
- Thermal
- Visual
- Vibration
- Space and furniture
- User posture
- Health hazards
- Protective clothing and equipment

Organizational Environment
- Work practices
- Assistance
- Interruptions
- Management and communications structure
- Computer use policy
- Organizational aims
- Industrial relations
- Job characteristics

This approach could be useful when designing an AT system, as it presents service providers with an understanding of the factors affecting usability of technology and, more importantly, a structure for evaluating the effectiveness of the AT system.

Human-centered approaches have also been used to improve device design, and the acceptability and usability of technologies.[26] Unfortunately, because of a paucity of research and development funding as well as a legacy of the rehabilitation model, AT is often designed without a sound understanding of the wants and desires of the users or contexts in which they are to be used.[38] It is not surprising that the appeal and usability of these products are often wanting.

Mainstream models of technology acquisition and implementation have explored the difficulties encountered with the introduction of new technologies into the workplace. Problems with implementation of technology have been identified at different levels, such as the individual, the work group, and the organizational level.[30] Models such as the Attributional Model of Reactions to Information Technologies (AMRIT)[30] have sought to explain individual capabilities and the user's capacity to determine the usefulness of technology. The AMRIT proposes that "the introduction of a new technology, along with other external environmental and intrapersonal influences combined with prior success or failure at tasks involving information technology, evokes causal attributions" (p. 315).[30] In this instance, attribution is drawn from attributional theory[55] and relates to the characteristics the user ascribes to the technology, based on generalizations from prior experience. These attributions reflect the expectations the user has regarding the outcomes for future performance with use of the technology and affect the user's affective and behavioral reactions to use of technology.[30] This model promotes a dynamic, interactive view of the variables and sees the interaction between the user and the technology as ongoing and constantly evolving. The model suggests that the user's attributions of the technology are formed and evolve before, during, and after AT is implemented.

Martinko and colleagues emphasized the influence of prior experience on the perception of information technologies and claim sufficient empirical evidence is available to support the contention that negative prior experiences with technology are related to the rejection of technology.[30] Additionally, the perceived usefulness and ease of use of the technology are important variables in assigning attributions, particularly when the technology is central to task performance. External influences also affect the acceptance of technology. The performance and expectations of others in the environment influence the degree of acceptance the individual demonstrates for the technology.

AMRIT shifts the focus from the individual and his predisposition to using technology to the ongoing interaction between the user and the technology. It proposes that prior experience, user expectations, external influences, and technology characteristics all influence the user's perception of the usefulness of the technology. AMRIT also suggests that negative experiences or perceptions of technology have a significant impact on the user's ability to accept or use the technology. Similarly, the usefulness of the technology and ease of use perceived by the users are important considerations in estimating the potential of the device.

AMRIT provides a sound foundation for examining variables that affect the acceptance of assistive devices. AMRIT has not been developed in the context of disability service provision and, as such, views the technology user as an active participant in the technology system. This model seeks to promote technology acceptance through appropriate application of the technology. The AMRIT presents a range of intervention strategies that promote acceptance of technology. Strategies suggested prior to the introduction of technology are: associating the technology with prior successful experiences; pretraining, which provides explicit levels of usage success; implementation plans that eliminate early failures and ensure early successes; screening users for technology-related attributions and expectancies; and involving users in system design. Intervention strategies post-introduction of technology are counseling to provide users with alternative attributional frameworks and opportunities for modeling successful users, providing successful images to cue facilitative user behavior, and redesigning technology systems to achieve positive attributions and expectations. Clearly this model—and the research associated with it—have much to offer AT professionals and their understanding of technology implementation.

SUMMARY

Models that guide AT practice have evolved from its foundation in the rehabilitation model through needs-based procedural models to models dedicated to the application of AT, such as the HAAT and MPT models. Each of these models defines our scope of concern and the nature of the services we offer. They influence the way in which AT users are perceived by service providers, how their needs are determined, and the interventions used. In this chapter, these models were reviewed in light of the social model of disability and their capacity to support client-centered practice. Mainstream models of technology application also were examined to determine their value in the selection and application of assistive technologies.

References

1. Bailey RW: *Human Performance Engineering.* Englewood Cliffs, NJ, Prentice Hall, 1989.
2. Bain BK, Leger D: *Assistive Technology: An Interdisciplinary Approach.* New York, Churchill Livingstone, 1997.
3. Barnes C, Mercer G (eds): *Breaking the Mould? An Introduction to Doing Disability Research.* Leeds, England, The Disability Press, 1997.
4. Batavia AI, Hammer GS: Toward the Development of Consumer-Based Criteria for the Evaluation of Assistive Devices. *J Rehabil Res Development* 27(4):425-436, 1990.
5. Baum CM: Achieving effectiveness with a client-centered approach: a person-environment interaction, in Gray DB, Quatrano LA, Lieberman ML (eds): *Designing and Using Assistive Technology.* Baltimore, Paul H. Brookes, 1998.
6. Bazinet G: Assistive technology, in Karan OC, Greenspan S (eds): *Community Rehabilitation Services for People with Disabilities.* Boston, Butterworth-Heinemann, 1995.
7. Brooks NA: Models for understanding rehabilitation and assistive technology, in Gray DB, Quatrano LA, Lieberman ML (eds): *Designing and Using Assistive Technology: The Human Perspective.* Baltimore, Paul H. Brookes, 1998.
8. Brooks NA: Users' responses to assistive devices for physical disability. *Social Sci Med* 32(12):1417-1424, 1991.
9. Butterworth J, Kiernan WE: Access to employment for all individuals: legislative, systems and service delivery issues, in Lehr DH, Brown F (eds): *People with Disabilities Who Challenge the System.* Baltimore, Paul H. Brookes, 1996.

10. Chadwick A: Rights on a wrong wheel: the dangers of a medical approach to civil rights, *Austral Disabil Rev* 2:40-59, 1995.

11. Cook A, Hussey S: *Assistive Technologies: Principles and Practice*, ed 2. St. Louis, Mosby, 2002.

12. Covington GA: Cultural and environmental barriers to assistive technology, in Gray DB, Quatrano LA, Lieberman ML (eds): *Designing and Using Assistive Technology: The Human Perspective*. Baltimore, Paul H. Brookes, 1998.

13. Cushman LA, Scherer MJ: Measuring the relationship of assistive technology use, functional status over time, and consumer-therapist perceptions of ATs. *Assistive Technol* 8:103-109, 1996.

14. Day H, Jutai JW: Measuring the psychosocial impact on assistive devices: the PAIDS. *Can J Rehabil* 9:159-168, 1996.

15. Demers L, Weiss-Lambrou R, Ska B: The Quebec User Evaluation of Satisfaction with assistive Technology (QUEST2.0): an overview and recent progress. *Technol Disabil* 14:101-105, 2002.

16. Dewsbury G, Clarke K, Randall D, et al: The anti-social model of disability. *Disabil Soc* 19(2):145-158, 2004.

17. Enders A: *Technology for life in a new disability paradigm. Keynote Presentation.* Paper presented at the Australian Conference on Technology for People with Disabilities, Sydney, September 28-30, 1999.

18. Fearing VG, Clark J: Individuals in context: a practical guide to client-centered practice. Thorofare, NJ, Slack, Inc., 2000.

19. Garber S, Gregorio T: Upper extremity assistive devices: assessment of use by spinal cord injured patients with quadriplegia. *Am J Occup Ther* 44(2):126-131, 1990.

20. Hocking C: Function or feelings: factors in abandonment of assistive devices. *Technol Disabil* 11:3-11, 1999.

21. Krefting LH: The use of conceptual models in clinical practice. *Can J Occup Ther* 52(4):173-178, 1985.

22. Law M: *Client-centered occupational therapy*. Thorofare, NJ, Slack, Inc., 1998.

23. Law M, Baptiste S, Carswell A, et al: *Canadian Occupational Performance Measure*, ed 2. Toronto, Canadian Association of Occupational Therapists, 1994.

24. Lenker JA: Professional education programs in rehabilitation engineering and assistive technology. *Technol Disabil* 9:37-48, 1998.

25. Lenker JA, Paquet VL: A new conceptual model for assistive technology outcomes research and practice. *Assistive Technol* 15:1-15, 2003.

26. Maguire M: Methods to support human-centered design. *Int J Human-Computer Studies* 55:587-634, 2001.

27. Mann WC, Hurren D, Tomita M: Comparison of assistive device use and needs of home-based older persons with different impairments. *Am J Occup Ther* 47(11):980-987, 1993.

28. Mann WC, Lane JP: *Assistive Technology for Persons with Disabilities*, ed 2. Bethesda, MD, American Occupational Therapy Association, 1995.

29. Mann WC, Tomita M: Perspectives on assistive devices among elderly persons with disabilities. *Technol Disabil* 9:119-148, 1998.

30. Martinko MJ, Henry JW, Zmud RW: Attributional explanation of individual resistance to the introduction of information technologies in the workplace. *Behavior Information Technol* 15:313-330, 1996.

31. Nochajski SM, Oddo CR: Technology in the workplace, in Mann WC, Lane JP (eds): *Assistive Technology for People with Disabilities*, ed 2. Bethesda, MD, AOTA, 1995.

32. Nochajski SM, Oddo C, Beaver K: Technology and transition: tools for success. *Technol Disabil* 11:93-101, 1999.

33. Oliver R: *The politics of disablement*. London, Macmillan, 1990.

34. Pedretti LW: Occupational performance: a model for practice in physical dysfunction, in Pedretti LW (ed): *Occupational Therapy: Practice Skills for Physical Dysfunction*, ed 4. St. Louis, Mosby, 1996.

35. Phillips B: Technology abandonment from the consumer point of view. *NARIC Quarterly* 3(2-3):4-91, 1993.

36. Phillips B, Zhao H: Predictors of assistive technology abandonment. *Assistive Technol* 5:36-45, 1993.

37. Post KM: The promise of assistive technology. *Am J Occup Ther* 47(11):965-967, 1993.

38. Poulson D, Richardson S: USERfit: a framework for user centered design in Assistive Technology. *Technol Disabil* 9:163-171, 1998.

39. Reed K: Theory and frame of reference, in Neistadt ME, Crepeau EB (eds): *Willard and Spackman's Occupational Therapy*. Philadelphia, Lippincott-Raven, 1998.

40. Reed K, Sanderson SN: *Concepts of Occupational Therapy*. Philadelphia, Lippincott, Williams & Wilkins, 1999.

41. Rogers JC, Holm MB: Assistive technology device use in patients with rheumatic disease: a literature review. *Am J Occup Ther* 46(2):120-127, 1992.

42. Scherer MJ: *Living in a State of Stuck: How Assistive Technology Impacts the Lives of People with Disabilities*, ed 3. Cambridge, MA, Brookline Books, 2000.

43. Scherer MJ: *Living in a State of Stuck: How Assistive Technology Impacts the Lives of People with Disabilities*, ed 4. Cambridge, MA, Brookline Books, 2005.

43b. Scherer MJ, Sax C, Vanbeirvliet A, Cushman LA, Scherer JV: Predictors of assistive technlogy use: the importance of personal and psychosocial factors. *Disabil Rehabil* 27(21):1321-1331, 2005.

44. Scherer MJ: The impact of assistive technology on the lives of people with disabilities, in Gray DB, Quatrano LA, Lieberman ML (eds): *Designing and Using Assistive Technology: The Human Perspective*. Baltimore, Paul H. Brookes, 1998.

45. Scherer MJ, Vitaliti LT: Functional approach to technological factors and their assessment in rehabilitation, in Dittmar SS, Gresham GE (eds): *Functional Assessment and Outcome Measures for the Health Rehabilitation Professionals*. Gaithersburg, MD, Aspen, 1997.

46. Seidel AC: Theories derived from rehabilitation perspectives, in Neistadt ME, Crepeau EB (eds): *Willard and Spackman's Occupational Therapy*. Philadelphia, Lippincott-Raven, 1998.

47. Smith RO: Measuring the outcomes of assistive technology: challenge and innovation. *Assistive Technol* 8:71-81, 1996.

48. Spencer JC: Tools or baggage? Alternative meanings of assistive technology, in Gray DB, Quatrano LA, Lieberman ML (eds): *Designing and Using Assistive Technology: The Human Perspective*. Baltimore, Paul H. Brookes, 1998.

49. Sprigle S, Abdelhamied A: The relationship between ability measures and assistive technology selection, design and use, in Gray DB, Quatrano LA, Lieberman ML (eds): *Designing and Using Assistive Technology: The Human Perspective*. Baltimore, Paul H. Brookes, 1998.

50. Steinfeld E, Angelo J: Adaptive work placement: a "horizontal" model. *Technol Disabil* 1(4):1-10, 1992.

51. Symms J, Ross D: Hierarchy of Assistive Technology. Paper presented at the RESNA Conference, Long Beach, Calif, 1991.

52. Uniform Data System for Medical Rehabilitation (UDS): *Functional Independence Measure*, version 5.1. Buffalo, NY, Buffalo General Hospital, State University of New York, 1997.

53. Verbrugge LM, Rennert C, Madans JH: The great efficacy of personal and equipment assistance in reducing disability. *Am J Public Health* 87:384-392, 1997.

54. Vincent C, Morin G: L'Utilisation ou non des aides techniques: comparaison d'un modeleamericain aux besoins de la realite quebecoise. *Can J Occup Ther* 66(2):92-101, 1999.

55. Weiner B: An attributional theory of achievement-motivation and emotion. *Psychological Rev* 92(4):548-573, 1985.

56. World Health Organization: *International Classification of Function, Disability and Health: ICF*. Geneva, WHO, 2001.

57. World Health Organization: The International Classification of Impairments, Disabilities and Handicaps (ICIDH). Geneva, WHO, 1980.

CHAPTER 3

Consumer-Centered Process for Technology Acquisition and Use

■ "Key to this process is recognizing and building on the expertise of the consumer as his or her own long-term 'technologist.'"[9]

On the face of it, providing assistive technology services seems simple.[8] There is an ever-increasing array of technologies designed to help people with disabilities undertake activities in which they were previously unable to participate. However, the bewildering range of technologies and fragmented services make it difficult for people to identify suitable devices and locate useful information and expertise. Assistive technology (AT) users, especially those with limited experience of assistive technologies, can quickly feel overwhelmed and ill equipped to make informed decisions. Without experience of the process and an understanding of what is involved, consumers find it difficult to retain control of the process, let alone direct it. Service providers, particularly those new to the field, also find it difficult to navigate the process. Dealing with the complexities of the technology and the process often means that it is difficult for them to appreciate that the users' needs extend beyond their limited contact with a specific service. As noted in Chapter 2, traditional practice approaches also make it a challenge for service providers to work in a consumer-centered way during their transient encounter with the AT user.

This chapter examines the process of selecting and using technology from the consumer's perspective. The first part of this chapter provides an overview of the steps in the process of technology acquisition and use as proposed in the literature. It draws from these to present a comprehensive understanding of the process AT users undertake when selecting and using technology. Each step of the process will be discussed in turn with a view to understanding these from a consumer's perspective. The resources required by AT users throughout this process will then be discussed. The objectives of this part are to (1) examine a number of procedural models proposed in the literature, (2) consider the experiences of AT users throughout the process, (3) outline the stages involved in acquiring and using technology in the workplace, and (4) detail the resources required by users for each of these stages from a consumer-centered perspective. The second part of this chapter will describe the details of the research study undertaken by the authors, which examines AT users' experiences of the process of technology acquisition and use in the workplace. The results of this study are discussed in depth in Chapters 4 to 8 of this book.

▒ EXISTING PROCEDURAL MODELS FOR TECHNOLOGY ACQUISITION AND USE

As indicated in Chapter 2, procedural models detail the process for addressing issues. These may be closely aligned with a conceptual model—for example, the Human Activity Assistive Technology Model (HAAT)[4]—or may be independent of a conceptual model. A number of procedural models have been presented in the literature that outline a series of stages involved in selecting and using technology (Table 3-1). Each of these models varies in terms of the scope, focus, and detail they provide. Because procedural models are developed primarily to guide practice, the context in which the author works often defines the scope of the model. Models designed to enhance AT service provision frequently address the selection phase of the process.[16] Models designed to assist the application of technology define the steps required for the successful implementation of technology.[4] Some models, which seek to provide a comprehensive view of the process, overview the steps involved in selecting and using technology.[1]

▒ OVERVIEW OF STEPS IN THE PROCESS

Envisioning Possibilities

A review of the stages proposed in the literature indicates that there are a number of steps in the process of technology acquisition and implementation. The process begins with a person envisioning what is possible and the potential that technology offers him.[1] Sometimes people come to the process with this vision; however, often it evolves slowly throughout the process. Our vision for the future is largely affected by our perception of ourselves and what we are capable of, our hope for what may be possible, and our understanding of what others have achieved. Throughout the device selection process, many service providers focus on developing a realistic understanding of the AT user's capabilities. This is often achieved by assessing the person's "naked" abilities—that is, what they are physically able to do without devices or assistance. Although this provides a baseline of capacities, it does little by way of creating a vision of possibilities. This approach also reinforces deficits at a time when people are trying to build on their capacities and develop an understanding of how they can be enabled to participate in society. The evolution of technology, on the other hand, continues to provide people with hope that technology can enable them to fulfill their aspirations.

With an understanding of technological developments and access to an ever-expanding range of technologic possibilities, people with disabilities can broaden their horizons and extend their vision of what they can do. However "success has more to do with people than machines" (p. 12).[1] People constantly extend themselves through creativity and determination and provide motivation to others to follow their dreams. Many people with disabilities have surpassed the expectations of professionals to attend university, run their own business, and become active members of the community. It is these role models and success stories that inspire people with disabilities to create a vision of what is possible and a new life story for themselves. Service providers need to embrace people's visions of what they want to be able to do and provide them with information on technologies

TABLE 3-1

Proposed Stages of Technology Acquisition and Implementation

STAGES OF TECHNOLOGY ACQUISITION AND USE	ALLIANCE FOR TECHNOLOGY ACCESS[1]	BAIN AND LEGER[2]	COOK AND HUSSEY[4]	KELKER AND HOLT[11]	NOCHAJSKI AND ODDO[16]	SCHERER AND GALVIN[24]	SPRIGLE AND ABDELHAMIED[25]
Identifying the Right Technology	Visioning possibilities, Setting goals		Referral and intake		Referral	Establish goals/expectations	
			Needs identification	Be realistic about child's capabilities and needs	Assessment	Assess need for no-, low-, or high-tech device	Identifying the user's needs
			Skills evaluation	Get a multidisciplinary evaluation			Measuring functional abilities
		Identifying the consumer's abilities	Identifying task requirements				Describing functional tasks
		Identifying the tasks	Reviewing environmental demands			Match person and technology	Comparing abilities to task demands
		Identifying present and future environment					Determining whether a device is indicated
			Identify device characteristics				Establishing device criteria

TABLE 3-1 (cont'd)

	ALLIANCE FOR TECHNOLOGY ACCESS[1]	BAIN AND LEGER[2]	COOK AND HUSSEY[4]	KELKER AND HOLT[11]	NOCHAJSKI AND ODDO[16]	SCHERER AND GALVIN[24]	SPRIGLE AND ABDELHAMIED[25]
	Reviewing technology tools	Identifying possible devices		Solution circle			
	Identifying local resources and supports						
	Developing a funding strategy						
		Evaluating the interface between the consumer and ATD	Recommendations and report	Evaluate the assistive technology			
		Selecting the ATD by all team members					
	Selecting equipment					Select	Selecting or designing a device
	Buying equipment				Procuring equipment		
Introducing Assistive Technology			Order and setup Delivery and fitting			Fit	

TABLE 3-1

(cont'd)

	AUTHORS						
	ALLIANCE FOR TECHNOLOGY ACCESS[1]	BAIN AND LEGER[2]	COOK AND HUSSEY[4]	KELKER AND HOLT[11]	NOCHAJSKI AND ODDO[16]	SCHERER AND GALVIN[24]	SPRIGLE AND ABDELHAMIED[25]
Optimizing Assistive Technology Use	Developing expertise—learning and training	Training the consumer to use and maintain the ATD	Training	Training of user and significant others	Training	Train person for AT use	
Ensuring Ongoing Use of Assistive Technology	Sharing your skills	Documenting the evaluation process Periodically reevaluating all parts of the AT system	Maintenance and repair Follow-along Reevaluation	Repair and maintenance Insurance Follow-up Reevaluation Monitoring—noting skills improvement Aware of upgrades	Maintenance and repair of device Monitoring for continued use of devices	Assess/evaluate outcomes according to goals/expectations	Evaluating AT intervention effectiveness

that can enable them to realize this vision. Alternatively, if the person has not yet developed a vision of what is possible, service providers need to assist them to imagine what is possible by providing information on what technology can offer, as well as contact with AT users who are using technology to achieve their goals.[3]

Accessing an Assistive Technology Service

Many service providers see the process of device selection and implementation as beginning from the point of referral to the AT service. However, for the AT user the journey begins well before the initial contact with a service provider and is likely to extend well beyond their encounter with any particular service. In order to make use of the services available, people with disabilities must first be aware that technology can offer them something and that there are services to assist them in selecting and implementing technology. It is often assumed that people are aware of the technologic possibilities and existing resources and are then able to procure a referral to these.[1,24] Many people who could benefit from technology may not even be aware of the possibilities or where they can access information or expertise on options. For this reason we may ask how AT service providers can reach out to these people and provide them with ready access to the information and expertise they require to explore technology options.

People who access AT services generally self-refer; alternatively, they are referred by other sources such as friends, other service providers, employers, or third-party payers.[16] Once contact is made, services gather preliminary information to determine if the facility is able to provide the necessary services and if the person is eligible to receive services based on the service's funding criteria. If there is no match between the AT user's requirements and the services provided, then the user needs to be referred to a more suitable service.[4] Alternatively, if the service is able to assist the AT user, the nature and extent of the services need to be clearly articulated.

Service providers need to assist the user and other stakeholders to understand what the process of selecting and implementing technology involves and identify the aspects of the process to which they can contribute. For example, some services are primarily focused on identifying potential technology options, whereas others are responsible for securing appropriate funding, providing training, or setting up and maintaining the technology. It is therefore important to identify what other services or providers need to be engaged to ensure the user is supported throughout the process. For example, if the service being accessed is primarily focused on identifying suitable technologies, then the AT user needs to be informed about accessing funding for the device and how to gain access to training and support for effective implementation.

Establishing Goals and Expectations

Before the potential of technology can be explored, it is necessary to examine the person's need and desire for technology.[24] Technology should not be seen as the panacea for all problems, but rather its relative benefits should be considered in conjunction with other alternatives, such as using an alternative strategy. Information is gathered about the person's preferences, past experiences, and expectations of technology to explore whether they are open to the use of technology and able to manage it. In addition, the capacity of the milieu/ environments to accept and support the technology also requires consideration.[24] Some consumers are likely to have a very clear and specific purpose for their technology,[25] yet others may require assistance to develop and articulate their goals.[22] Service providers, with their understanding of technologies, their features, and trade-offs can often assist by providing the consumer with an understanding of what is possible.[25] Collaboration with other stakeholders (e.g., family, teachers, therapists, or employers) may also assist in developing specific goals and expectations of the technology.[4,16,24,25]

Many therapists use informal interviews to develop an understanding of a person's goals; however, structured processes offered by tools such as Goal Attainment Scaling (GAS)[15] and the Canadian Occupational Performance Measure (COPM)[13] can assist in developing a detailed understanding of the person's current level of performance and priority goals. In addition, these tools provide a mechanism for evaluating the effectiveness of the technology in addressing the person's goals. The Matching Person Technology (MPT) assessment process has been specifically designed to examine a person's technology needs, and the forms provide a structure for exploring goals, preferences, and the person's view of technology.[22] Once the person's overall goals have been determined, it is possible to identify the range of technologies that have the potential to assist in achieving these goals. For example, a goal of returning to work would indicate that a person with a spinal injury would need to explore computer and mobility technology.

Identifying Specific Requirements

The next stage of the process focuses on establishing the user's specific requirements.[2,4,11,25] A good definition of the user's requirements is needed to identify the best technology.[25] Traditionally AT service providers have been initially concerned with details such as the person's age, size, weight, among others,[25] to determine the appropriate dimensions of the device, for example, a wheelchair. In addition, some procedural models have focused on evaluating the person's specific skills and abilities.[2,4,25] However, as noted previously, it is not always necessary for the AT service provider to undertake a detailed analysis of the user's "naked" abilities to determine the functional requirements of technology.

Some users with established impairments are able to provide a reliable report of their functional capacities, which would be sufficient to enable the service provider to identify the type of technology options to explore without the need for further assessment. Similarly, children often have teams whose members can provide detailed reports of the child's current skills and capacities. The AT service provider will, however, need access to information about the person's impairments, abilities, and past experience with technology[4] to understand the person's specific capacities and requirements. This allows the user and the service provider to identify the type of technology best suited to the individual's level of function and the specific features required by the individual to use the technology effectively.

It is not always possible to predict how well someone will manage a piece of technology from this information alone. People can often use alternative methods to perform the same action.[25] It is, therefore, necessary to observe the person using technology to accurately evaluate the suitability of a device.[25] For this reason, functional assessment of the user's ability to use devices to perform specific tasks is likely to give the service provider and the user a much clearer understanding of the client's capacities and requirements than a detailed evaluation of functional capacities.

Defining Task Requirements

With service providers being focused primarily on identifying the person's abilities and impairments, little attention has been given to defining the task requirements of the technology. This shift in focus from the *person and their abilities* to what it is they want to be *able to do is* very important. In line with the social model of disability, it requires service providers to move from fitting the technology to the person to configuring technology to meet the person's activity requirements. In this way service providers can align themselves more closely to the user's goals and ensure that the technology provides users with the social and psychological freedoms they seek.[23]

A number of models highlight the need to describe and analyze the activities to be performed using the technology.[2,4,24] Cook and Hussey identify activity as a fundamental element of the HAAT model.[4] Valued activities are identified by examining the person's life roles and identifying the activities that contribute to these roles. Considering activities at this global level often results in general goal identification, such as improved communication, mobility, and computer use similar to those established at the goal identification stage of the process. Increasingly, with the development of integrated technologies, it is important to examine how activities relate to each other in a life role rather than considering each activity goal as a discrete entity.

For example, at work someone may need to undertake data entry, read documents, make appointments, dispatch letters, and communicate over the phone. By defining each task to be undertaken, the user can determine the specific functions they require of technology and consider how technology might be integrated to enable him to participate in all these activities effectively. It is necessary also to examine activities at a more discrete level; that is, identifying each task involved in the activity so that barriers to activity engagement or task performance can be examined at each stage. For example, a user may want to use a computer for word processing, navigating the Internet, drawing, and data entry, all of which require varying input speed and control. By determining the requirements of each task, a range of input devices can be explored to determine which are best suited to each task.

Review of the Application Environments

Over the past few decades, there has been increasing awareness of the environment and how it can enable or limit participation. It is important to consider the settings in which the person is likely to be using the technology; that is, at home, school, workplace, or out in the community,[2,4] acknowledging those they are currently in as well as future application environments.[2] AT service providers should aim to extend the range of environments the AT users can operate in, rather than limiting them to a specified environment. The physical aspects of the environment also require careful consideration. Technologies need to be able to manage the topography, temperature, climate, sound, and lighting conditions of the application environments[2,4] and interface with existing electronic systems in the environment.[4] The milieu of psychological, social, and cultural aspects of the application environment is also critical to the success of technologies.[4,22] Technology needs to be acceptable to the user and others in the environment, as well as able to be supported in the application environment. Furthermore the technology should enable the AT user to participate equitably and meet the expectations of others in the environment.

Establishing Device Criteria

Once it is determined that technology has the potential to meet the person's goals,[4,25] device criteria/characteristics need to be established.[1,2,11] This stage of the process requires that the person's specific requirements and the demands of the activity or activities and application environment(s) are detailed so that the specific features of the technology can be identified.[4] The user's goals would determine the nature of technology explored while their preferences would indicate the style of device in which the user might be interested. The user's experience with technology often dictates the level of sophistication he will be comfortable with while his skills and abilities will determine the interfaces and programming requirements. See Table 3-2 for an analysis of the technology characteristics based on the person's requirements.

Outlining the range of activities and tasks to be performed (both now and in the near future) will assist in determining the specific features and functions required of the technology system. See Table 3-3 for an analysis of the technology characteristics dictated by the nature of the activities to be undertaken. This may result in a number of devices being integrated to provide the necessary functions or one device being configured to meet the range of demands. The nature of the tasks to be undertaken will determine also the input, storage, programming, and output specifications of the technology.

By examining the range of environments in which the technology is to be used and the nature of these environments, the AT user and service provider can determine (1) the impact of the environment on the technology, (2) the impact of the technology on the environment, (3) existing or proposed technology with which the devices need to work, and (4) the support available or required to support the technology. Table 3-4 provides an analysis of the technology characteristics as defined by the application environments.

As each area of the AT system is considered, it will become apparent that some features are compatible with requirements in other areas while some may contradict other requirements. At this stage it is necessary to discuss priorities

TABLE 3-2

Technology Characteristics Based on the Person's Requirements

PERSON	TECHNOLOGY CHARACTERISTICS
Goal: To return to office work	Computer technology with modern office software
Preference: Sleek, modern look	Black casing and flat screen
Experience: Word processing experience in Microsoft Word 95	Consider Microsoft family of software
Skills and abilities: limited vision, limited ROM, strength and endurance in upper limb, mobilizes in power wheelchair	Standard keyboard layout, enlarged visual output, light touch keyboard/voice input, reduced keyboard size/trackball, word prediction capabilities, able to be positioned easily (e.g., monitor arm and adjustable workstation)

TABLE 3-3

Technology Characteristics Based on the Requirements of the Activities to Be Undertaken

ACTIVITY	TECHNOLOGY CHARACTERISTICS
Word processing	Keyboard voice entry (additional RAM)
Data entry: numbers	Separate numeric keypad
Navigating desktop and Internet environment	Mouse or alternative
Answer the phone	Headset, computer-based phone answering software
Need to man the reception area for 2 hours a day	Duplicate or portable system for reception area
Emailing and managing household finances at home	Compatible/duplicate system at home

TABLE 3-4

Technology Characteristics as Defined by the Application Environments

ENVIRONMENT	TECHNOLOGY CHARACTERISTICS
Open office environment	Quiet operation
Floor to ceiling glass windows	Discrete device
Strips of fluoro lights with diffusers running length of ceiling	Glare screen for enlarged monitor
Networked environment running on Windows environment	Windows-compatible software and devices
High output expected	Efficient system
Funding limited	Cost-effective solution
Funding dedicated for workplace accommodation	Devices to meet workplace requirements

so that they can be appropriately weighted when evaluating the usefulness of potential options.

Identifying Potential Devices

The range of available mainstream and specialized technologies is ever-expanding, and it is becoming increasingly difficult to distinguish between them.[1] It is useful, therefore, to have a sound understanding of what mainstream technologies can offer before exploring the value of specialized technologies. The Internet provides easy access to a wealth of information, such as supplier catalogues and online databases, that allows users and service providers to be aware of the range of devices available; however, without some understanding of or experience with the technology, it is difficult to determine which devices are worthy of further exploration. Some AT users find this stage of the process overwhelming and find it useful to explore local resources and develop a "circle of support"[1] to assist them to locate and navigate the diverse information systems and identify technologies that have the capacity to meet their requirements. Resource people can include those with general technology expertise, assistive technology service providers and information services, AT suppliers, friends, and other AT users. Each of these people brings a different perspective and understanding of technology and its benefits, and they are worthy of consultation.

Developing a Funding Strategy

At this time it is also necessary to develop a funding strategy.[1,2,11] Because there are limited established funding sources for assistive technology, AT users need to be very resourceful and persistent to secure adequate funds for the technology.[1] Furthermore, AT users are likely to encounter administrative and bureaucratic obstacles when investigating their funding options. It is, therefore, essential that they develop an understanding of the funding schemes available and their funding criteria, or that they use their circle of support to assist in identifying a suitable funding source and navigate the administrative processes to achieve a good outcome. The circle of support also can be useful in assisting the AT user to identify additional expenses associated with the specific purchase.[11] For example, a number of costs can be anticipated, including the costs of upgrading the computer or workstation so that it can accommodate the new technologies, training, ongoing maintenance and repairs, and factoring in the costs of upgrades.[11]

Trialing and Evaluating the Suitability of Technologies

The suitability of devices is then determined by examining the interface between the consumer and device[2,4] and evaluating how well each meets the technology requirements determined earlier in the process.[1,2,4,24,25] Trialing the device is imperative. This enables the user to review the aesthetics, comfort, and usability of the device, and the service provider to examine the fit between the user and the interfaces. Together the AT user, service provider, and other stakeholders can determine how well each device meets the criteria and discuss the relative merits of each option.

Purchasing Technology

After the device is selected,[1,16] it is then purchased.[4] For most AT users, ongoing technical assistance is critical.[1] It is important to consider the experience and reliability of the supplier when deciding where to purchase the technology. So that there is no confusion as to who holds the responsibility for attending to issues, it is useful, where possible, to purchase all required equipment and accessories from one vendor. It is also useful to question the vendor about the range of ongoing maintenance he provides; if he provides training, installation, and upgrade support; and the cost of these services.[1] Other AT users and service providers are also useful resources for examining the experience and reliability of suppliers.

Setting Up and Fitting Technology

Assistive technologies frequently need to be set up by someone with appropriate expertise[4,24] to ensure they are operating as intended and are integrated with the work setting technologies.[16] In addition the technology needs to be fitted to the specific requirements of the user.[1,2,4,11,16,24]

Training

Training is fundamental to effective use of technologies.[4,11,16] Without adequate training, it is likely that the technology will be abandoned.[4] Frequently, specialist training is required to equip the AT user to use her technology effectively. It is necessary, therefore, to anticipate the user's training requirements in the funding application so that she can acquire the skills and knowledge to operate the technology in the work environment.[4] Training is also most effective if well-defined objectives are established.[4] AT users need to develop "operational competence"[4]; that is, to be able to turn the device on and off, know how to adjust the various features of the device, understand the maintenance requirements, and troubleshoot problems they are likely to encounter in using the device. In addition, users require "strategies competence,"[4] which enables them to use the device to perform specific tasks. Operational training can be provided soon after delivery of the device, whereas strategic training is most effective when the user is "on-the-job"[16] and familiar with the range of tasks for which she will be using the device. It is important to be aware that it can be challenging for AT users to develop the skills required to carry out work tasks while developing skills in using their new device.[16] By providing AT users with access to ongoing training support, they can continue to develop skills after they have established basic competencies.

Maintenance and Repair Follow-Up

Service providers are often tempted to think that the process is complete once the technologies are in place; however, this marks the beginning of the implementation process for the AT user.[4] First, it is essential that the technologies are maintained if they are to be effective.[16] AT users need to know how to maintain the device and who to contact when it is in need of repair.[11] Once again, these are ongoing costs that need to be considered when costing the technology.[16]

Insurance is an other important consideration when examining the ongoing costs associated with technology.[11]

Monitoring and Evaluation

Many models then advocate that the process be documented[4,11,24,25] and that an evaluation of the effectiveness of the AT or outcome be undertaken.[2,4] In addition, some models advocate periodic reevaluation[11,16,24] and on-going monitoring of use.[1] These models, in particular the HAAT model,[4] acknowledge that there are likely to be changes that influence the ongoing effectiveness of the acquired technology. First, the AT user's skills will continue to develop, or his condition may change, necessitating a change in technology. Second, changes to the tasks the user performs may require that the technology be reviewed. Third, changes to other technologies, such as a computer upgrade, may result in incompatibilities. Finally, there may be changes in the setting that place additional demands on the technology that had not been anticipated. Because of the number of issues that are encountered throughout this process, one model acknowledged the importance of sharing skills and knowledge acquired throughout the process,[1] so that others can benefit from users with experience in selecting and using the technology. Another model also highlighted the importance of monitoring technology upgrades in the area,[11] so that the user can benefit from important technologic developments.

◼ USING A PROCEDURAL MODEL TO GUIDE THE PROCESS

When a process is undertaken, it is important that it be congruent with the basic assumptions underpinning our conceptual system. For example, if working from the HAAT model,[4] the process should allow the fit between the person, activities, technology, and environment to be examined and have structures in place to address the ongoing changes in the AT system. In addition, the social model of disability would be reflected in identifying the activities and environments the person wishes to engage in, ensuring that barriers are removed from the environment and that strategies are put in place to enable ongoing participation. Within the conceptual and procedural models, the person should also be recognized as having unique needs and coping strategies. Furthermore, for a process to be client-centered, it must empower the user to direct the process, ensure he has the respect of the service providers, and grant him autonomy in making decisions. This requires that the process focus on the person's concerns and that these are addressed using existing strategies and supports. In addition, services need to be accessible[9] and responsive to the user.[2,4,16,24,25] Rather than viewing the process from the perspective of the service provider and what services can or should be provided, we need to understand the experience of users as they explore their technology options and seek to use them effectively, as well as the resources and strategies they find useful in this process.

It is important to note that most of these steps[2,16,25] have been proposed by service providers to guide other providers through the process. Many are written from the providers' perspective and are concerned with the clinical support required to advance a user through device selection and use. These models vary in terms of the degree to which they acknowledge the role of the user in the process. Some are concerned with measuring the user's abilities and prescribing the most appropriate solution.[4,24] Others outline processes that acknowledge the uniqueness of each user and the application environments and use language that is more inclusive of the user.[18,21] Recent research has found that a lack of consideration of the user leads to abandonment or nonuse of devices,[7] and that involving the user during the process positively influences device use.[26] However, the degree to which users are involved in the process depends on their understanding of what is involved and the opportunities afforded them by the service provider and the approach/process used. It is important that users be aware of what the process entails if they are to be meaningfully involved or work collaboratively with service providers.

A key issue is that service providers often have only transient contact with users and are not always available to address issues that arise on a day-to-day basis or a few years down the track. Service providers may be restricted in terms of what part of the process they can contribute to or how long they can provide support, whereas AT users need to be aware of the whole process and what is involved at each stage, and be empowered to direct the process to achieve effective long-term solutions and be their own "long-term technologists."[9] Alliance for Technology Access[1] and Kelker and Holt[11] outline the process from a user's perspective, recognizing that users need to be able to envision possibilities[21] before they even seek information or support. These models acknowledge that users have the ability to explore options independently and make use of supports within their own communities. They recognize that users ultimately hold the responsibility for recognizing their need for technology, accessing and using resources and supports, and ensuring that the technology continues to meet their needs. If users are to direct the process and make informed decisions, it is important that they understand what is possible, what the process involves, the range of resources available, and how they can make good use of technology long term.

▨ CONSUMER-CENTERED APPROACH TO SELECTING AND USING TECHNOLOGY

When talking with AT users about the process of selecting and using technology in the workplace, users do not talk about identifying their needs and evaluating outcomes. The process they use to select and use technology is not dissimilar to the way many of us choose a new car or computer, except that for AT users, the choices are limited and the resources are more scattered.[9] Although each of us has his own personal style for making decisions about new purchases, we essentially go through a similar process. The quality of the outcome is dependent on us having a clear idea of our requirements, knowledge of the options available (or the availability of suitable expertise to assist us in identifying what is available) and taking care to match our requirements with the available options. To heighten our sensitivity to the experience of the AT consumer, take some time to reflect on a recent purchase, the process you used to select it, and the resources and the strategies you used to optimize your use of this equipment.

Reflect on the last time you bought a new computer or car.

- How did you go about it?
- What was your vision of this car/computer; that is, what is important about a car/computer for you (e.g., efficiency, speed, the way it looks)?
- What do you want to be able to do with your car/computer?
- Who are the primary user/s? What additional considerations did you make for others?
- What were your specific requirements in relation to (1) person (i.e., your preferences, experience, skill, and interests), (2) activities (What do you want to be able to do with it?), and (3) environment (Where will you be using it? Who else has a stake in this?)
- What important features were you looking for in the car/computer?
- How did you find out what kind of cars/computers are available?
- Who did you have/need to support you in this process?
- What experience did you need with this car/computer prior to purchase?
- How did your budget affect what and where you purchase the car/computer?
- After you purchased the car/computer, (1) what additional adjustments or supports did you need to ensure you used it effectively and that it continued to work well? (2) How did you learn to get the most out of your computer/car? And (3) what do you do to ensure the computer/car continues to work effectively for you?

Reflecting on a recent technology purchase, it becomes clear that you benefited from previous experience with technology and an understanding of what was possible to envisage what you wanted. Depending on your knowledge or experience, you probably used a range of resources (e.g., talking with others, reading reviews, and seeking the opinions of a range of sales people) to gather information and reach your decision. In addition, it is likely that there were many competing factors to consider and compromises required. You may also have had to consider other people in the household, facilities in the environment, and your future needs to ensure the purchase had good long-term potential. Furthermore, you would have familiarized yourself with the technology, adjusted it to your preferences, developed your skills in using it, and established what was required to keep it in good working order. Unless you had a parent or kindly friend or relative to walk you through the process, it is likely that you had to identify and use a range of resources and supports throughout this process. The steps you undertook and the resources you used are likely to be similar to those outlined in Table 3-5.

It can be seen that the steps in selecting a new computer or car are very similar to the steps identified in the literature for AT users when selecting and using technology. There is one notable difference between the steps outlined here and those identified for AT acquisition and implementation, namely, accessing a specialized assessment service. The range of resources people generally use when selecting and using a new purchase are many and varied. In reality this is

TABLE 3-5

Steps in the Process of Selecting and Using Technology and Resources Required

STEPS IN THE PROCESS	RESOURCES USED
Visioning possibilities	General media, seeing what others use, talking with people with similar goals/experience
Establishing goals/expectations	Talking things over with friends or people with experience or expertise
Identifying specific requirements	Examining and appraising personal skills and experience through self-reflection or testing or seeking expert advice
Defining required features	Expert advice, talking with friend, reflecting on personal goals and experience
Information on potential technologies and resources	Information systems (formal and informal): experts, Internet, directories, reading relevant literature, friends, and advertisements
Locating local resources and supports; develop a funding strategy	Seek recommendations from experts and friends, search local directories
Trialing and evaluating options	Display rooms, demonstration models with access to friends and experts to weigh relative benefits
Purchase device	Manufacturer and supplier
Integrate with other technologies	Supplier, expert, or friends
Customize device to personal requirements	Supplier, expert, or friends
Learn to use device	Attend a course, read manual, ask a friend with experience, experiment
Maintenance and repair	Maintenance and repair services
Insurance	Supplier, expert, or friend
Review ongoing suitability	Expert, friend, self-reflection
Upgrade the technology as the need arises	Information on new technologies and recent advances in current technologies

also true for AT users; however, service poviders do not have a very deep understanding of the user's experience of the process, the barriers they experience, or the strategies they make use of to progress them through the process of selecting and using technology. Much of the literature to date has focused on the process from the service provider's perspective, outlining procedures for delivering services. There has been very limited exploration of the realities experienced by AT users in general and none to date that has focused specifically on integrating technology into the workplace. Given the very specific expectations and demands that exist in varied workplaces, it is vital that service providers have a deep understanding of the challenges that users experience.

The next part of this chapter will describe the AT user study that forms the basis of the remaining chapters in this book. In this part, the study participants and details of the methodology used to gain a deep understanding of consumer perspectives in selecting and using technology in the workplace will be described.

The AT User Study

Before undertaking this study a reference group was formed to provide a forum for discussing procedural decisions, monitoring decision-making, and discussing analysis and interpretation of the data. This group consisted of two of the researchers, a service provider and a consumer who was also an active advocate for people with disabilities. The National Disability Research Grant (NDRG) and the Centre of National Research on Disability (CONROD) provided funding for this research and requested utilization of a reference group with consumer involvement.

Participants

The 26 AT users who contributed to the research referred to in the rest of this book were recruited through information disseminated through newsletters and mailouts to a broad range of disability organizations and service providers in Queensland, Australia. Ten employers and 10 coworkers also provided input. The AT users had a range of congenital and acquired conditions, including visual impairment, cerebral palsy, rheumatoid arthritis, multiple sclerosis, and spinal cord injury. A detailed description of the participants can be found in Table 3-6. The technology users worked in paid open employment from 10 to 40 hours per week. They ranged in age from approximately 18 to 55 years. Four of the technology users were women and 22 were men.

In terms of geographic location, 15 technology users lived and worked in a metropolitan region, five worked in nonmetropolitan regions within 3 hours of a major city, and six lived and worked in rural towns. Three participants were self-employed, two were contact workers, nine participants worked in small community organizations, seven worked in local or state government departments, and five were employed by federal government departments. With regard to their types of jobs, eight described themselves as working in administration and five as managers or program coordinators. Four participants ran a business, five worked in education or research positions, two in computer programming, and two as professionals (e.g., engineer and lawyer).

The technology users made use of a range of low-tech and highly sophisticated technologies. These included a combination of wrist supports, access software, specialized keyboards, on-screen keyboards, text to speech software, and voice recognition software. Details of types of technology used can be found in Table 3-6. Some participants used very specific technology for specific tasks, whereas others used a range of technology for multiple applications. They had a wide range of experience with mainstream technology. Some participants required support to operate within specific applications, whereas others could problem-solve independently and embraced new technology enthusiastically. Similarly, some participants were unaware of the existence of specialized technology information and resources or were supported by service providers to access specific resources. However, others actively sought and used an extensive range of resources.

TABLE 3-6

Characteristics of Participants in Research Study

INITIALS	DISABILITY	WORK TASKS	AT USED
A	C5-6 spinal injury	Word processing PowerPoint	Typing splints Trackball Manual wheelchair
B	Rheumatoid arthritis–some manipulation difficulties	Word processing Email/web Telephoning	Compact keyboard/voice recognition Graphic tablet mouse Hands-free phone Electric wheelchair
C	C4-5 spinal injury	Word processing Email/web Telephoning	Naturally Speaking Marble trackerball Hands-free phone Electric wheelchair
D	Spinal muscular atrophy	Word processing Spreadsheet Email/web Telephoning	On-screen keyboard Mouthstick Hands-free phone Electric wheelchair
E	Amputation arm/shoulder	Word processing Telephoning Driving	Compact keyboard Headset for phone Adaptations
F	Spinal injury from birth	Word processing telephoning	Access Pack Head set Electric wheelchair
G	Vision impairment from birth: severe short-sightedness	Reading and writing Data entry and management Microfiche	Closed-circuit TV Text enlarger Enlarged screen
H	Overuse syndrome– manipulation difficulties	Word processing Desktop publishing, database entry	Naturally speaking Kensington Trac ball
I	C4-5 spinal injury	Data entry telephoning	Access Pack, Keywiz, macros Mouth/headstick Phone with headset Electric wheelchair
J	Cerebral palsy–walks with limp Manipulation difficulties	Word processing and Excel Desktop publishing and PowerPoint Email Phone	Tried Dragon Dictate Hands-free phone
K	C4-5 spinal injury	Word processing Spreadsheets Email telephone	Dragon Dictate Classic Typing sticks Trackball Mounted handset Electric wheelchair
L	Acquired vision impairment (1985)– peripheral shadows	Reading Word processing Email/web	Kurzweil Personal Reader Screen reader Text enlarger

TABLE 3-6

(cont'd)

INITIALS	DISABILITY	WORK TASKS	AT USED
M	Cerebral palsy– difficulty communicating using speech	Word processing Telephoning	Electric wheelchair Headpointer Hands-free phone
N	C3 spinal injury	Text entry Email/web Telephone	Electric wheelchair Dragon Dictate 2.5 Trackball Mouthstick Hands-free phone
O	Cerebral palsy– difficulty communicating using speech	Windows 95 Invoicing program	Electric/manual wheelchair Keyguard Joystick mouse
P	Cerebral palsy–mild mobility and manipulation difficulties	Spreadsheets Word processing Telephoning	Wrist supports Word prediction, Access software Standard telephone
Q	C5-6 spinal injury	Accounting package Phone	Electric wheelchair Typing splint Access Pack Omnikey Ultra Dragon Dictate(start)
R	Multiple sclerosis– severe manipulation difficulties	Accounting package MYOB Word processing Web and email Phone	Electric wheelchair Naturally Speaking Phone through computer
S	Vision impairment– severe short-sightedness	Data entry Word processing/ spreadsheet Desktop publishing/ email	Closed-circuit TV Zoomtext
T	Vision impairment– total loss of vision	Reading Word processing, Excel/email/web Notetaking Listening to taped manuals/docs Message taker/Item and doc marker	Brailler/scanner/tape recorder Screen reader Braillite Business memo device Perkins Brailler'

Sampling

Purposive sampling was used to select information-rich cases. The study aimed to explore the varied experiences of people with disabilities who used AT to work in open employment. Specifically, maximum variation and criterion sampling were used to identify key informants.[17] Maximum variation sampling was used to include a diverse range of people in the research. As mentioned previously, extensive measures were undertaken to recruit participants to represent people throughout the working age range with a range of congenital and acquired disabilities and both genders. People working in a range of job types and in a variety of work environments were also sought. Maximum variation sampling is designed to capture common patterns that cut across variations, as well as detailed descriptions of unique and diverse experiences.[17] Exploring the experiences of a range of people from a variety of settings also enhances the ability to generalize the findings.[10]

Criterion sampling also ensured that the study focused on people using AT to carry out essential work tasks in open employment. During the initial telephone conversation, the investigator asked the technology user for demographic background information such as age and job title, as well as information about their work-related technology. This enabled the investigator to ascertain whether the person met the inclusion criteria. Inclusion criteria included AT users who (1) had an impairment that affected their ability to carry out work tasks, (2) worked in paid employment a minimum of 10 hours per week, and (3) used at least one type of technology (assistive or mainstream computer technology) within the work environment.

It was agreed that no more than 50% of participants would be accepted at the suggestion of the Queensland Independent Living Centre (ILC-Qld) Technology Service, in order to also obtain information from people who did not use a specialist AT Information Service. Although initially an inclusion criterion of a minimum of 20 hours or more per week employment was considered, this excluded a number of people who had useful information to share. It was also found from initial phone contacts that, depending on the severity of disabilities, people who used AT in the workplace often worked parttime. So the criterion was adjusted to accommodate this on advice from the reference group.

Once a range of participants had been located, snowballing or chain sampling was then used to maximize the number of participants. After a number of months of recontacting service providers, informants who had already been identified were being repeatedly nominated by a range of people. According to Patton,[17] this is an expected result of snowballing or chain sampling and suggested that the sampling procedure had identified relevant key informants.

Procedure

After ethical clearance for the conduct of the project was gained through the Behavioural and Social Sciences Ethical Review Committee at The University of Queensland, participants were initially recruited via mail to disability organizations, service providers, and employer groups. Disability associations included groups representing impairments such as acquired brain injury, cerebral palsy, spinal injuries, and neurologic conditions. Services included rehabilitation, disability, and employment services. Information about the study was circulated through newsletters to members, through e-mails to service providers, and via staff meetings and memorandums. Interested technology users were asked to contact the researcher by telephone. Several technology users contacted the researcher directly; however, most participants were first nominated by service providers. These service providers passed on the study information to the potential informants who telephoned the investigator. Participants who met the inclusion criteria were invited to nominate a suitable time to be interviewed.

Data Collection

A series of open-ended questions were developed by the reference group on the basis of their experience, the literature, and the objectives of the study. The interview protocol was piloted with one AT consumer, and minor modifications to the sequence and wording of questions were made on the basis of this person's experience with the interview. The interview questions are provided in Box 3-1. All interviews were completed in the person's usual work environment. Permission was also sought to photograph the technology user at his or her desk/workplace. These photos provided the investigator with visual information about the person's workstation. If a coworker or employer was nominated, a suitable time for this independent interview was scheduled. Coworkers or employers were asked similar questions, with some modifications as identified in Box 3-1. Interviews ranged from 1 to 2 hours in length. All interviews were audiotaped and transcribed verbatim after the interviews. A field diary was kept by the investigator about the work site, technology used, and any other relevant observations, reactions, or reflections after each interview. The use of such a diary provides a means of taking into account personal reactions to the visit and possible bias in interpretation.

Member checking was used to strengthen the credibility of data.[14] After the interviews were transcribed and coded, the participants were sent an individual summary of the interview and key themes identified by the researchers in their particular interview. They were asked to read these summaries, add any further comments to them, and finally sign and return them to acknowledge their agreement with the summary and interpretations of the content of their interview. All participants signed and returned these.

Analysis of Data

The interview transcripts were the main source of data. Thematic analysis of the content of interviews was undertaken using QSR NUD*IST Version 4 software to assist with data management. Content analysis is the systematic examination of text and field notes by identifying and grouping themes and coding, classifying, and developing categories.[19] Because independent assessment of transcripts adds to the reliability of the data analysis,[19] interview transcripts were read independently by the first and third authors and one of the other members of the reference group, each of whom identified recurring key words and emerging themes. Two investigators at a time discussed their individual classification of transcripts in terms of recurring key words and clustered these into emergent themes. Discussion ensued to develop consensus between all investigators as to the identification of issues and themes.

BOX 3-1
Interview Questions

Objectives of the Interview
- To understand the process of decision-making
- To understand how technology is being used in the workplace: the types of technology and tasks for which they are used
- To understand whether technology is effective in meeting the user's needs in the workplace, and if not, why not
- To understand what has helped with the use of technology to perform work tasks
- To understand what things have hindered the use of technology to perform work tasks
- To understand what processes are in place to address changes in the workplace, tasks, technology, and individual's function

Questions
Key questions are italicized, and probe questions are also listed to elicit further information where the participant does not provide it.

1. *Tell me how you came to decide on what technology you needed for work?*
   How did you determine what you needed?
   How did you know what was available?
   Did you get to trial a number of devices?
   Who made the final decision as to what you needed?
2. *Who was involved?*
   What resources did you use in identifying your technology needs?
   How much did they know about technology?
   How much did they know about helping to set it up for you?
   Did you use an ATP or information service? Why not?
   How useful was it?
   How long did this take?
3. *What did you think about the process?*
   How useful were these resources?
   What did you feel about the process?
   What were the best features?
   If you were to do it again, what would you change?
4. *Who funded your technology needs?*
   Did the funding available affect the technology choices available to you?
5. *What type of equipment are you using?*
   Why did you choose those devices?
   What other options did you explore?
   Did you have an opportunity to trial them before you purchased them?
   How did you determine that they were appropriate to your needs?
6. *What tasks are you using them for?*
7. *How effective is the technology in assisting you to perform your work tasks?*
   Do you have any difficulties performing these tasks using the technology?
   Are you managing your work tasks efficiently?
   What would you need to do to improve your efficiency?

BOX 3-1
(cont'd)

Do you have problems with recurring errors, things taking too long to complete?
What would you like to change about the technology?
What other technologies have you used in the past?
How effective were they in helping you perform your work tasks?
Why did you stop using them?
How did you come to have them?

8. *Are there other technologies that would assist you with your work?*
   Are there activities or tasks you still find difficult that could be improved with the use of technology?
   Are you aware of any technologies to assist you with these?
   If there were, how would you go about finding out what you needed, getting it, setting it up to use at work, and learning how to use it?

9. *How do you feel about using technology?*
   Have you had much previous experience?
   Do you use it anywhere else? How?

10. *What would help you to feel at ease using technology?*

11. *How have you set the technology up to suit your specific needs?*
    Have you had to adjust the positioning of the equipment?
    Have you fiddled with the features of the technology to make them suit you better?
    Are you comfortable when you are using the equipment?
    Do you think the technology is working well for you? Would you like to change anything?

12. *How did you learn to use the technology?*
    How long did this take?
    Who or what assisted you in learning to use the technology?
    Do you feel confident in using the technology?
    Can you think of anything that would have helped develop confidence in using the technology?

13. *How did you learn to use it to perform your work tasks?*
    Who or what assisted you in learning to use the technology to perform work tasks?

14. *Tell me how the technology was set up in the workplace?*
    Who set it up?
    How long did this take?
    Who assisted you in setting up the technology?

15. *Who supports it when there are problems?*
    Do you have any ongoing compatibility or maintenance issues?
    Who assists you in resolving these?

16. *What would happen if there were changes in the computer platform, network, work tasks, office location, workstation, or your condition?*
    What happens when work practices change or computers are upgraded?
    Who assists you in resolving difficulties encountered?
    Is there someone who has been involved in the implementation of your technology? Who is he or she?
    Can we speak with this person about the technology?

BOX 3-1
(cont'd)

17. *Does the technology affect your coworkers in any way?*
    Has it changed the way you work?
    Are there any jobs that you used to delegate that you can now do yourself?
    Has it created any obstacles in the workplace for others?
    Are there any technologies you use that others envy?
18. *Has there been an occasion when you were unable to do your job because the technology let you down?*
    What processes did you use to resolve the issue?
    Did you put anything in place to deal with this issue in the future?
19. *Has there been an occasion when you were able to use the technology unexpectedly to perform a task?*
    Were you able to integrate that into your day-to-day work activities?

Interview Questions for the Employer: Integration of Technology into the Workplace

What kind of accommodations need to be made in the workplace to accommodate the person's technologic needs? How much IT support is required to establish the equipment and to keep it operational?

What did you need to do to assist the person to use AT in the work environment?

How long did this take?

What or who assisted you in this process?

What difficulties have you encountered?

What have you learned from these?

Are you happy with the way things are working?

How could it be improved?

Do you have any ongoing compatibility or maintenance issues?

Who assists you in resolving these issues?

What happens when the office is changed around, work practices change, or computers are upgraded?

How would you go about resolving difficulties encountered?

What advice would you give another employer/supervisor in a similar situation?

Interview Questions for the Coworker: Integration of Technology into the Workplace

What kind of accommodations need to be made in the workplace to accommodate the person's technologic needs? How much support is required to establish the equipment and to keep it operational?

Does having a person use AT in the workplace have any impact on you?

What, if any, involvement have you had with the person using AT in the workplace?

What, if any, support have you had in this process?

What difficulties have you encountered?

What have you learned from these?

Are you happy with the way things are working?

How could it be improved?

What advice would you give another coworker in a similar situation?

The data were initially organized into units related to the progressive stages of integrating technology, such as statements related to identifying technology, acquiring technology, and integration of technology and skill development, as well as statements related to user approach to the process, technology experience of the participant, and the nature of the work environment. Within each of these units, statements were further coded to gather detailed information about the participants' experiences at each stage of the process. Within these statements, themes began to emerge about the barriers participants encountered, as well as the strategies and supports they found effective.

Cross-case analysis was also undertaken to explore the heterogeneity of the group of participants. This form of analysis enables cases to be roughly compared and assists in synthesizing interactions between phenomena.[10,17] During the analysis, it was noted that participants' experiences and approaches varied. This raised questions about the level of support required by each AT user and, more importantly, who was most at risk of not accessing an appropriate level of support. A number of parameters were identified, such as use of resources, level of interest in exploring options independently, access to funding, cost of technology, technical problems encountered, access to IT support, learning experience, level of technology use, support in the workplace, and willingness to self-advocate. These variables were examined to understand the diverse experiences of the group. For example, it was noted that while some participants did not use specialist resources to find out about technology or only accessed resources they encountered, others accessed a service provider who alerted them to a number of resources. Alternatively, other participants actively explored the resources available independently. This analysis provided an understanding of the diversity of AT user experiences and the complex interactions between the person, the AT, and the environment.

Rigor

In order for research to be accepted as being worthwhile, it is essential that the quality of the investigation is maintained. The term *rigor* is used to refer to strategies that are used to ensure the trustworthiness or merit of a qualitative inquiry.[12] Rigor is concerned with the credibility of the research and acknowledging the influence of subjectivity on research design, data collection and analysis, and focusing on minimizing its effect.[20]

Rice and Ezzy proposed that rigor should be maintained consistently throughout the research process, and described five ways in which it should be addressed.[20] These are as follows: first, when the research question is being explored, theoretical rigor is required to ensure that the research design is appropriate. Second, procedural rigor is used during data collection to enable clear documentation of methodologic and analytic decisions. During data analysis, a range of practices, such as triangulation, are used to promote the third form of rigor known as interpretive rigor. Evaluative rigor, the fourth form, addresses issues related to the ethics and political aspects of the research. Finally, by documenting the researcher's stance and reporting on the role of the researcher, issues of reflexivity also are addressed. Strategies used to address rigor throughout this study will now be described.

Theoretical Rigor

Qualitative researchers approach research with a basic set of beliefs or assumptions that guide their investigation.[5] Cresswell proposed that there are five philosophical assumptions that are central to all qualitative studies: ontologic, epistemologic, axiologic, rhetorical, and methodologic.[5] The ontologic assumption proposes that reality is subjective and multiple. In a phenomenologic study such as this, the researcher is charged with reporting on the diverse perspectives provided by the participants of the phenomena being explored. A diverse range of people in a variety of workplaces was sought for this study to explore the range of experiences people have with integrating technology into the workplace. The use of purposive sampling also increases the transferability of the findings.[12] By capturing a heterogeneous group and describing central themes, maximum variation sampling provides information on common patterns that emerge from this diversity of experience that generalize more readily to the larger group.[17]

The second philosophical assumption, epistemologic assumption, highlights the relationship between the perspectives of the researcher and the participants. It acknowledges the need to decrease the distance between the researcher and the participants to understand the participants' experiences. In qualitative research the researcher is viewed as an active learner who relates the story from the participants' viewpoint, details their experiences, and builds a complex, holistic picture of the phenomena.[5] By seeking to understand the AT users' personal experiences in using their technology in the workplace, the researcher viewed herself as an active learner in this research. The axiologic assumption calls for researchers to acknowledge their own values and biases. Phenomenologic inquiries require researchers to set aside or bracket these prejudgments so that they can be open and receptive to what the participants are saying and not impose an a priori hypothesis on the experience. Identifying the assumptions and values that the researcher brings to a study also has been identified as being important in developing the rigor of an investigation. Details of the researcher's stance throughout this study will be discussed further in rigorous reflexivity.

Qualitative research values the personal experiences of the participants and therefore uses personal and literary narratives to tell the story. This rhetorical assumption places importance on the terms and language used by the participants to relate their experience. The methodologic assumption provides a foundation for the inductive logic used in analyzing the narratives and generating codes and themes. This study sought to explore the uniqueness of the human experience and to describe the range of those experiences to improve the dependability of the data.[12] In this study the codes and themes emerged from the participants' stories, and the research questions evolved further as the researcher became more familiar with the range of experiences AT users had in integrating their technology into the workplace.

Although the theory on which this research is based is primarily interpretive phenomenology, some aspects of postmodernism have influenced the authors' stance. The marginalization of people with disabilities in society and the changing politico-social climate in the workplace has had a significant impact on the availability of work for people with disabilities and the climate of acceptance in the workplace. Although this investigation was not shaped by this theoretical perspective, the authors are well aware of the impact of antidiscrimination legislation on the experiences of AT users and the implications of this research on society's perceptions of AT users. Although this research is not based on grounded theory, the potential for it to provide an understanding of the complexities of integrating AT into the workplace on which theories of service provision can be further developed cannot be ignored. The value of alternative theoretical perspectives in adding to the depth and potential of this research has been actively explored and would provide further rigor through theory triangulation.

Methodologic Rigor

By providing a detailed account of how the research was conducted and how decisions were made, methodologic rigor can be maintained. The reference group also provided a means of monitoring procedures and discussing decisions. In addition the researcher met regularly with an experienced qualitative researcher to discuss concerns and perceptions, and to reflect on the rigor of the methodology. The use of QSR NUD*IST Version 4 software, a computer-based system for the storage and analysis of transcripts, also assisted in tracking transcripts and noting the evolution of the analysis.

Two methods of triangulation, namely data and investigator triangulation, have been identified by Denzin and Lincoln[6] and Krefting[12] as a means of attending to the validity of the design and analysis in qualitative research. These two methods of triangulation were used to strengthen this study. Triangulation of the data was achieved by using researcher observation of the technology user in their work environment, photographs of the user at his or her workstation, and the interview data. The observations provided information about the way in which participants were using technology, and the photographs provided information about the place of the technology in the work environment. The coworker and/or employer perspectives were used in this study to provide contextual information to help interpret the informants' meaning. Investigator triangulation was achieved by using three of the members of the reference group in the analysis of the transcripts.

Interpretive Rigor

Descriptive data about the participants and the accompanying detail in the results and discussion were provided earlier to assist the reader in determining the transferability or applicability of this research to other contexts.[12] The trustworthiness of this research is assisted by the use of substantial quotes from the primary texts to support the analysis. Truth value also addresses whether there is confidence in the representation of the multiple realities of the participants.[12] Accuracy was sought in this study by the use of member checking. Participants were sent a copy of the transcript, as well as a summary of the major issues raised in the interview for them to check for accuracy of the interpretation of the interview. A field diary also provided the authors with an opportunity to discuss evolving perceptions with one another. As discussed previously, two of the authors were involved with reading and analyzing the transcripts and identifying emerging themes. These themes were then discussed, and consensus was reached on the terms to be used and their definitions. Presence of an AT user on the reference group also assisted interpretation.

Evaluative Rigor

This research received ethical clearance for The University of Queensland, Behavioural and Social Sciences Ethical Clearance Review Committee. This Committee requires researchers to attend to ethical considerations before commencement, such as potential for harm, procedures for addressing unanticipated issues, informed consent, confidentiality, and data security of research projects.

Rigorous Reflexivity

Rigorous reflexivity examines the role of the researcher in the process. Denzin and Lincoln proposed that "qualitative researchers self-consciously draw upon their own experiences as a resource in their own inquiries" (p. xi).[6] As such, the researchers are biographically situated in the research and draw on their own experience to interpret the data.[6] This, they proposed, results in the researcher adopting a particular view of the people being studied, in this case the AT users. For further details on the researchers' perspectives, see "Authors' Stance" in the Preface.

A field journal was used to record feelings, thoughts, and ideas throughout the research process. Periodically these were discussed to provide an opportunity to reflect on values and assumptions and to discuss whether these were impacting on the data collection and analysis.

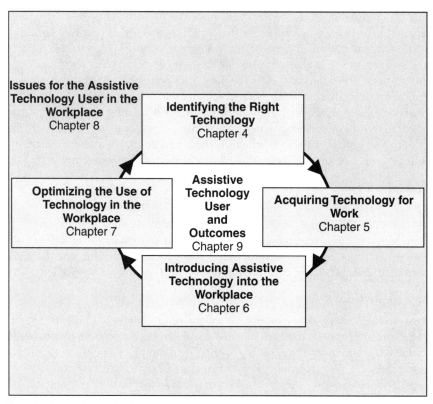

FIGURE 3-1 ▨ Stages in the AT process.

▨ EXPERIENCE OF ASSISTIVE TECHNOLOGY USERS

This study demonstrated that AT users have similar experiences and concerns when they are investigating the potential of technology. That is, the steps outlined previously in Table 3-5 would be almost identical for selecting any major piece of technology. AT users are concerned with understanding how technology can assist them, identifying the right technology, acquiring it and introducing it into the workplace, setting it up to meet their specific requirements, learning to use it, managing issues related to their technology in the work environment, and, finally, optimizing their use of technology long term. Each stage of this process will be examined in the subsequent chapters of this book in light of the AT users' experiences. These stages are outlined in Figure 3-1.

In the following chapters each stage of the process will be examined and discussed from the perspective of AT users. Direct quotations from the participants in the study will be italicized for clarity. The quotations leading into each subsequent chapter have been drawn from AT users involved in the study.

SUMMARY

The process of selecting and using technology involves many steps that have been variously described in the AT literature. However, if the needs of AT users are to be effectively met, it is important that the process is viewed from their perspective and that the steps they go through to select and use their technology are clearly identified. This ensures that appropriate resources are developed that empower users to address their ongoing technology needs. In an effort to understand more fully the experiences of AT users as they navigate this process, a qualitative study was undertaken.

The methodology of this study has been described in this chapter, and the results will be detailed and discussed in Chapters 4 to 8.

References

1. Alliance for Technology Access: *Computer and Web Resources for People with Disabilities.* Berkeley, Calif., Hunter House, 2005.
2. Bain BK, Leger D: *Assistive Technology: An Interdisciplinary Approach.* New York, Churchill Livingstone, 1997.
3. Baum CM: Achieving effectiveness with a client-centered approach: a person-environment interaction, in Gray DB, Quatrano LA, Lieberman ML (eds): *Designing and Using Assistive Technology.* Baltimore, Paul H. Brookes, 1998.
4. Cook A, Hussey S: *Assistive Technologies: Principles and Practice,* ed 2. St. Louis, Mosby, 2002.
5. Creswell JW: *Qualitative Inquiry and Research Design: Choosing among Five Traditions.* Thousand Oaks, Calif., Sage, 1998.
6. Denzin N, Lincoln Y: *Strategies of qualitative inquiry.* London, Sage, 1998.
7. Gage M: Re-engineering of health care: opportunity or threat for occupational therapists? *Can J Occup Ther* 62(4):197-207, 1995.
8. Galvin JC: Assistive technology: federal policy and practice since 1982. *Technol Disabil* 6:3-15, 1997.
9. Gradel K: Customer service: what is its place in assistive technology and employment services? *Vocational Rehabil* April:41-54, 1991.
10. Huberman AM, Miles MB: Data management and analysis methods, in Denzin NK, Lincoln YS (eds): *Collecting and Interpreting Qualitative Materials,* Thousand Oaks, Calif., Sage, 1998.
11. Kelker K, Holt R: *Family guide to assistive technology.* Cambridge, Mass, Brookline Books, 2000.
12. Krefting L: Rigor in qualitative research: the assessment of trustworthiness. *Am J Occup Ther* 45:214-222, 1991.
13. Law M, Baptiste S, Carswell A, et al: *Canadian Occupational Performance Measure,* ed 2. Toronto, Canadian Association of Occupational Therapists, 1994.
14. Lincoln YS, Guba EG: *Naturalistic Inquiry.* Newbury Park, Calif., Sage Publications, 1985.
15. Malec JF: Goal attainment scaling in rehabilitation. *Neuropsychological Rehabil* 9(3-4):253-275, 1999.
16. Nochajski SM, Oddo CR: Technology in the workplace, in Mann WC, Lane JP (eds): *Assistive Technology for People with Disabilities,* ed 2. Bethesda, Md., AOTA, 1995.
17. Patton MQ: *Qualitative Evaluation and Research Methods,* ed 2. Newberry Park, Calif., Sage Publications, 1990.

18. Phillips B, Zhao H: Predictors of assistive technology abandonment. *Assistive Technol* 5:36-45, 1993.
19. Pope C, Mays N: Research the parts other methods cannot reach: an introduction to qualitative research methods in health and health services research. *Br Med J* 311:42-45, 1995.
20. Rice P, Ezzy D: *Qualitative Research Methods: A Health Focus*. Melbourne, Australia, Oxford University Press, 1999.
21. Scherer MJ: *Living in a State of Stuck: How Assistive Technology Impacts the Lives of People with Disabilities*, ed 2. Cambridge, Mass., Brookline Books, 1993.
22. Scherer MJ: *Living in a State of Stuck: How Assistive Technology Impacts the Lives of People with Disabilities*, ed 3.Cambridge, Mass., Brookline Books, 2000.
23. Scherer MJ: The impact of assistive technology on the lives of people with disabilities, in Gray DB, Quatrano LA, Lieberman ML (eds): *Designing and Using Assistive Technology: The Human Perspective*. Baltimore, Paul H. Brookes, 1998.
24. Scherer MJ, Galvin JC: An outcomes perspective to quality pathways to the most appropriate technology, in Galvin JC, Scherer M (eds): *Evaluating, Selecting, and Using Appropriate Assistive Technology*. Gaithersburg, MD, Aspen, 1996.
25. Sprigle S, Abdelhamied A: The relationship between ability measures and assistive technology selection, design and use, in Gray DB, Quatrano LA, Lieberman ML (eds): *Designing and Using Assistive Technology: The Human Perspective*. Baltimore, Paul H. Brookes, 1998.
26. Wielandt PM, McKenna K, Tooth LR, et al: Post discharge use of bathing equipment prescribed by occupational therapists: what lessons to be learned? *Phys Occup Ther Geriatrics* 19(3):49-65, 2001.

CHAPTER 4

Identifying the Right Technology

> ▪ "The advancement in technology has continued to make me more independent and more efficient absolutely.... Just mainstream technology has helped a lot. Up until I broke my neck there were no computers so the potential business or work areas for people like myself were a lot more limited. So when computers became available they opened up a big area. Well with the advancements in technologies to do with that area it has just continued to make us more independent and more and more efficient."—AT Study Participant

To be part of the workforce, a person needs to be able to carry out work activities independently and efficiently. Although advances in mainstream technologies have provided more inclusive work environments, an ever-increasing array of assistive technologies (AT) is being developed that enable people with specific requirements to participate equitably in the workplace. But how do people find out about these technologies and decide which will best suit their needs? Identifying the right technology is the first stage in the complex process of choosing and integrating technology into the workplace (Figure 4-1).

Chapter 4 examines this first stage of the process of selecting and using technology in the workplace. It presents the first major section of results of the AT user study described in Chapter 3 and examines AT users' experiences regarding identification of the right technology. The second part of this chapter details recommendations for service providers emanating from consumers' experiences. The aims of this chapter are to examine (1) users' experiences of this stage of the process, (2) the issues consumers faced, (3) the strategies that enabled them to identify suitable technologies, (4) the range of information resources used, and (5) their contribution to the user's understanding of available options.

A number of themes emerged when AT users talked about their experience of identifying suitable technologies. These included (1) knowing what was technologically possible, (2) being aware of their needs, (3) finding out what was available, (4) individualized approaches to the process, (5) the importance of trialing devices, and (6) keeping up with technologic developments. These will now be described in turn.

▪ USER EXPERIENCES

Knowing What is Technologically Possible

Participants reported that they needed to be provided with a vision of what was possible in order to be inspired by the potential of technology. One participant expressed this clearly:

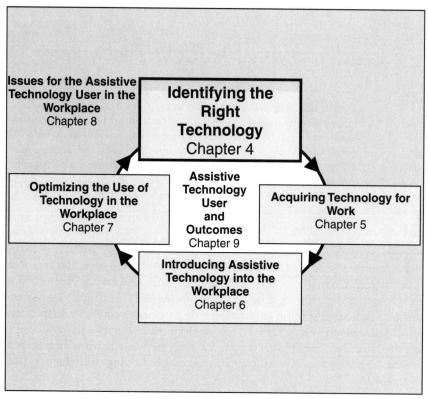

FIGURE 4-1 ■ Stages of choosing and integrating technology into the workplace.

Once I actually came in contact with the technology I could tell that it was exactly what I needed.

Employers also believed that it was important to fully understand the possibilities:

If people are not aware of the assistive technology and aids that people might access, then they're not going to be able to explore those with the particular employee. You need to have some sort of knowledge of all the possibilities.

A number of participants felt uninformed about what technology could offer. Without an awareness of what was possible, the participants reported that they had difficulty imagining how their work situation could be improved.

Those who did not have an awareness of available options often did not seek out possibilities. Employers also commented on the difficulties experienced by their employees when they were not aware of technologic possibilities:

Not a lot of information gets out; sometimes, it's not available for them. They say "I didn't know that was available, that I could use that." All of their lives they have been sort of struggling to do something and there it is; and they're not aware of it.

A number of participants stumbled upon their technology by accident. Finding out about solutions by chance was a source of frustration to some participants as illustrated in this quote:

With the headset, again because that was a fairly well-used piece of equipment at the Paraplegic and Quadriplegic Association, I was offered that as well which was really great but I wish I had known about that in my previous job. It would have made life much easier.

Even those who reported being computer literate still expressed uncertainty about how they could use technology to carry out their work tasks more effectively. Although some continued using their current technique, others referred the problem to computer literate friends in the hope that they could help. One participant said:

I didn't know what was going to be possible and he (computer literate friend) had the understanding. I told him that I needed something so I could use a mouse and he said he would look into it and see what he could find. So I didn't really picture anything in my mind.

Several spoke of the difficulty they experienced in identifying how technology could assist when they were not able to discuss possibilities with someone with similar needs. One stated: *You're naturally much more isolated in your needs I guess because you're often the only one around that has got those needs.* They felt that talking with someone with similar needs would have helped them become more aware of possibilities and to clarify their needs. The value of this exposure was confirmed by a participant who felt that seeing another person with a similar impairment using technology assisted him in identifying what he could use.

One gentleman who felt uninformed about alternative options was uncertain if he was using the best option. He commented: *I think... there might be a lot of other assistive technology out there that I haven't really looked at but I'm sure I could utilize.* People who were not aware of the range of technology possibilities often accepted the first option they encountered without evaluating whether it would meet their needs.

In summary, the importance of being able to envision technology and its positive impact was important to both employees and employers. It is important to get product information out to everyone in the workplace in a medium that is regularly accessed by potential users. The support of peer users is laudatory, and they, too, need to be kept regularly informed of product developments, especially how products may be beneficial in adapting to changing needs.

Awareness of Needs

Some participants commented that they experienced a decline in work performance or work-related health issues before they recognized that the issue required attention. One stated: *It puts me behind the eight ball in the sense that I have to wait...fall behind, before I realize that I need to change.* Participants tended to persist with current ineffective methods until there was a major problem such as persistent, severe pain or the risk of losing their job. One employer also noted that the user had held off using technology until the situation became critical. She stated:

As I understand it he (the participant) has been here (in the workplace) for some time and this type of equipment has been offered to him before. It has only been since he got the fright with the eye that he has finally taken that up. He realizes that he needs this type of equipment. I think he tries to just get by.

AT users reported that being unsure of what they needed made it difficult to explore potential technologies. For some, identifying needs was a matter of guesswork. One participant commented: *Well it was mainly trial and error; you tried something out and if you found it worked effectively, you used it.* Some participants took on new technologies at the suggestion of another technology user: *He suggested that I might like to try it...So we decided to give it a go.* For many participants the process was ad hoc rather than systematic.

A number of AT users highlighted the importance of having an understanding of their individual needs in identifying the best solution. One stated:

It's a bit more than knowing about the technology, knowing more about the person, about the disability too, because there's technology out there for all kinds of things, but you've got to match it to the right person.

Employers were aware how much they relied on the employee to identify his/her own needs prior to starting a job so that their technology requirements could be anticipated. One employer stated:

We needed to talk with him (the employee) about what he believed his individual needs were which was a bit difficult coming into a new job. So he had to try and work out what the job was going to be and identify his needs.

As a group, the participants with spinal cord injuries (SCI) appeared to be more certain about what they needed and, therefore, felt able to search for appropriate solutions. Seven of the 11 participants with SCI reported that they worked out what they needed independently. Some were able to anticipate their needs by thinking things through prior to commencing work, whereas others worked things out through experience, resolving issues as they arose. The AT users with SCI emphasized that it was essential to be clear about what you needed when exploring the technology. Participants who had a good understanding of their work tasks reported having a better understanding of their potential technology needs. One employer outlined a useful process for identifying needs and prioritizing technology purchases:

We actually looked at identifying what his job was and then deciding what he needed to use to get that job done. Once we knew what his tasks were going to be and the way that he would do them...we made a list of what we would really like to have and then we worked out what we could really afford to have.

The participants with other impairments, however, had variable experiences in attempting to identify their needs prior to exploration.

Although some participants required time in the job to determine their needs, others relied on accumulated work experience to delineate their needs. One person with vision impairment stated:

The basic skills and things that I've taught myself over many years as a blind person...and I just applied those to the new work environment.

Others drew on previous experience with technology to allow them to be much clearer about what they wanted from technology.

Some participants found the assistance from a service provider useful when identifying their needs. One participant noted how the service provider assisted him in analyzing his work tasks: *Well she came out here and said "Well okay; run through what you do." I sort of tried in as much detail as possible just to tell her.* Another appreciated having a professional to focus on the reality of his situation, *giving me real rather than unreal expectations of what I'm going to do.* Another participant valued the two-way process he had with the occupational therapist (OT) in identifying his needs. This extract from his transcript reflects his feelings:

> *We had a clear idea of it, because we conversed well, me and she (the service provider). She comes over and I explain and she gives me ideas, I give her ideas.*

Acknowledging individual preferences was also seen as being important. Not all the participants in this study readily embraced technology. One consumer preferred to keep his adaptations simple, as reflected in this statement: *I didn't know if I wanted a sophisticated program anyway.* Another issue for the participants was the *look* of the technology and its impact on how people viewed them as individuals. A number of participants commented on not wanting to look supported by technology or look *disabled*. One participant explained why she chose a scooter over an electric wheelchair in this statement: *Well for starters mostly because...it looks less disabled.* This view had an impact on the amount of technology they chose to use and their choice of technology.

AT users who had a good understanding of technology felt that service providers were most beneficial for people who are not able to work things out for themselves. However, one participant, who was well informed about technology, found it helpful to have an OT advise him on ergonomic and postural issues. He felt that this was more important than knowing about the technology available.

Some service providers were not only very helpful in assisting the user in identifying current needs, but were also able to anticipate future needs. One participant articulated this well:

> *We had to find out what was necessary for this position, but also what would be necessary if I moved on (to another job). What we ended up getting would be beneficial to me if I decided to find other work.*

Employers also noted the importance of considering the AT user's long-term needs. One employer articulated the value of this in the following quote:

> *I suppose that is one lesson we learned...that is, think about the future requirements of the technology, maybe get that up front.*

This allowed the user to make decisions that were more likely to withstand changes in the short-term and be of long-term benefit. As these employees will inevitably be long-term users of AT, they also need ongoing access to resources that can inform them of technologic developments which could be of benefit to them. One employer who provided a participant with contract work was aware of the need to keep abreast of technologic changes. He commented: *We have to upgrade; we have to advance in our technology as time goes on.*

In summary, an awareness of needs and available supports for those needs (e.g., technology, a personal assistant) go hand-in-hand. Each individual will have a different and unique perspective of what will likely work best. It is important to help them articulate their needs, as well as their preferences for how those needs can be effectively addressed.

▓ FINDING OUT WHAT WAS AVAILABLE
By Accident or through Own Resources

A number of the participants found out about technology by accident. One participant lamented:

> *It was word of mouth...if he (the doctor) wasn't using it (voice recognition technology), then I wouldn't have found out about it.*

Another participant commented: *You just had to be in the right place at the right time to find out about them.* Participants felt that it was often difficult to find out what existed because of the specialist nature, limited availability, and knowledge about AT.

Many felt constrained by having to rely on their own limited knowledge. One participant recalled:

> *But in the end all that did rely on my knowledge and what I was aware of, and because that was limited, even though it was a good positive process, really it fell down.*

One of the more computer-literate participants commented on the difficulties he encountered when exploring options with limited knowledge:

> *You don't always get the information you are looking for if you don't ask the right person the right question.*

Some found the process of finding out about technology manageable and even enjoyed investigating options and finding sources independently. One confident participant stated:

> *I go out and find out what's available and then we sit down and see how much we can spend.*

However, working independently did not always ensure that the most appropriate ATs were located. One participant commented:

> *I've always been probably too independent; wanting to do it myself and thinking I should be able to do it myself. Probably sometimes to my advantage and other times to my disadvantage or my detriment.*

Informal Contacts

Many of the participants reported using informal contacts to find out about technology. These included people with a disability in a related work area, contacts made through a disability group, or a personal friend with computer expertise. Some participants reported that informal contacts did not always have the right expertise, breadth of understanding, or knowledge of resources that could be accessed for further exploration. However, others commented that informal contacts were readily available, free, and could help them understand computer technology.

Suppliers and Specialist Resources

Those who used suppliers commented that their advice was often restricted to and biased by the range of equipment they sold. One stated:

> Of course I expected a fairly biased recommendation from some of those places but it was just a matter of sort of finding out what I could about prices and what people felt different ones could or couldn't do and seeing which way it all pointed.

Others maintained ongoing contact with suppliers and found them to be a useful resource.

Some participants did not know that special AT services existed. Despite having recently been through the process of identifying his technology, one participant remained unclear about the resources available. Without access to appropriate resources, some participants were denied the assistance they required. One participant took more than 5 years to access the support required to identify suitable technology. In the interview, he commented:

> So it was really only the last, say, 3 months that I've really got onto people that have helped me.

Some felt limited by their lack of access to experienced service providers. One participant recalled:

> There was no one who sat down and looked at the technology and said, "This is what you can do...this will be a help, how about trying this."

Most participants reported that they would have liked better access to information or specialist AT services. One participant noted that he would also like employment services to be more aware of the specialist information services and use them better.

Many learned about specialist resources during the process of identifying their technology needs. They commented that they would have liked to have known about them before they started their investigations so that they could have used them better. AT users who were aware of specialist services felt that they should have made better use of them.

> I suppose I should have gone to the (specialist AT service)...I think really (in hindsight) that possibly would be the only thing that I'd change.

Participants often found it difficult to use existing services due to time constraints. One participant who worked full-time was unable to investigate voice recognition technology due to time restrictions:

> I've known about Dragon (Dictate) for years and have never really decided to look into it until I was made redundant and had more time to do that.

Most participants who used a specialist AT information service felt that a central or specialist AT information service was the best way to access information about technology options. One participant, in particular, really valued the information he received from a specialist AT service. Another highlighted the benefits of having a service dedicated to understanding the technologic possibilities. He commented: *Someone who was up to date with what technology exists and could actually advise you on the possibilities.* Some participants felt that a specialist AT service offered more than information. The ability of staff to identify the individual's needs and explore an appropriate range of technology options was an important part of what was offered.

Those who received support from an employment rehabilitation service or disability organization were very happy with this support. It enabled them to locate resources quickly and reduced the stress on them to organize things. One user stated:

> *They were very helpful and very informative in getting back to me with all that stuff anyway, and basically just assisting me to work through processes, which was good.*

The participants found that these support services assisted them in identifying their needs, understanding current policies, and were also very resourceful in accessing funding and other relevant services. Several participants identified the support of service providers as the best part of the process. One person said:

> *They (the OTs) knew what they were doing and they were coming up with ideas, and once you think of something, they can look at it as well, adapt to a certain position that you may need. I didn't find it that hard with them so it went fairly easy...they've got it all on hand there and all the OTs go to courses and find out the latest stuff.*

Contact with Other Users

Some users highlighted the need to talk with someone with similar needs in preference to talking with a service provider or equipment supplier. One participant reflected:

> *If I had somebody in a similar situation to me that I could talk to who had been using the technology and get some ideas from them as to which was the best technology that would have suited us, I think that would have been easier than relying on somebody who had such a good understanding of the whole range to technologies, but had never lived in a wheelchair in an adapted household.*

A number of the participants were keen to have contact with other AT users during the selection process, and to benefit from their experience and knowledge of the technology. One commented on the benefit of this type of contact:

> *Especially the old timers cause they know a lot more than what we know...I'd end up wanting to talk to someone who's already got what I'm chasing.*

Others relied primarily on a user network to explore options as illustrated in this quote:

> *Some of it was just personal contacts that I had. Blind friends that I had or contacts that I had through, for instance, the blind computer user group.*

Another commented that it would also be most beneficial for technology to be demonstrated by someone with a disability who actually relied on it. He said:

> *If we could have people around who would be happy to show off what they're using and how effective it is, I think that would be very useful.*

For a number of participants, contact with other users was also one way that they kept up-to-date with technologic alternatives.

However, some participants were wary of relying solely on recommendations from other users. One participant highlighted his experience:

A mate of mine...said "I've got this fantastic program I think it will work for you". I could have gone out and bought that but he sort of gave me a copy and said "try it and..........". And I did. And it wasn't that easy, you know; it wasn't that good.

Although people may have similar impairments, their needs were often different. One participant noted:

I've spoken to other people who work in the workplace and who have visual disabilities and they're not actually using anything that is something that I could use.

Another participant commented on how his work demands differed from other people with similar impairments, which required him to work things out for himself through trial and error.

Internet

Although people were aware of the potential of the Internet to provide information about technology options, only a few participants reported using it to locate information about suitable options. Despite acknowledging the potential of the Internet to access information directly, one participant used a listserv for people with disabilities to request information on technology options rather than accessing online databases or Web sites about products. He commented:

Now compared to a few years ago, there is a lot more information readily available and, particularly on the Internet and things like that too, that's (the listserv) the best thing for me as far as just being able to search for information. It's wonderful.

Need to Use Range of Resources

Participants acknowledged the need to explore options widely. One participant commented: *If I were to do it again, I would be more prepared to inquire further and not accept the first one that I came across.* Participants needed to obtain information from a range of sources and to understand which information was most reliable. One participant noted: *It does pay to check out all options, not just accept what people say.* He also felt that, with experience, he had learned who was best to talk to. Some participants were able to explore technology options using a range of networks and resources. One participant felt that being well informed about options enabled him to make a good decision about the best technology for him.

Employers also valued the information gained from a range of sources, including talking with users of the technology. When searching for information on devices, one employer stated:

We contacted a real range of people; we contacted (a local information and advisory service)...*we contacted quite a few users, but I think that was our best source of information.*

In summary, there are myriad ways in which employees and employers find out about technology and, to many, the system seems disorganized and haphazard. Service providers and manufacturers can facilitate the information dissemination process by using a variety of means of promoting products and services.

Individualized Approaches to the Process

When talking with AT users, it became apparent that individuals differed in the range of resources they used and their level of understanding of technology options. Some were either not aware of the resources that existed or only accessed resources as they encountered them. Others had contact with service providers who assisted them in accessing relevant resources, or they actively sought out resources themselves. Their investigations resulted in some participants only being aware of the specific device they had encountered or the few that they trialed, whereas others were aware of all relevant options or had an active interest in continually exploring potential options.

One group of participants who enjoyed the process of exploring resources and technologies was aware of the current range of technologies and accessed information and expertise as required. Other participants were very active in exploring resources, but were not interested in developing an understanding of the full range of technology options, preferring to rely on expert professionals to identify the most appropriate technology. Another group was largely guided by service providers in using resources to find out about technology and identify the most appropriate option. Although these participants were aware of the specific options they explored, they were not aware of the full range of options available. A number of these participants did not have an active interest or a lot of experience with technology and were, therefore, very accepting of the advice given to them by service providers. These participants felt well supported during this experience, but they did not have a clear idea of the range of technologies and resources available to assist them in addressing their future needs. The last group of AT users was only aware of the specific resources and technologies they encountered in the process. Often they were unsure whether there were other technologies better suited to their current needs and felt ill equipped to review their technology needs. Participants with limited awareness of resources or who accessed limited resources were unaware of the range of technologies available to meet their current needs or the resources that could assist them in the process.

Opportunity to Trial Devices

Some participants did not trial equipment and were very happy with the application of the technology after purchase. However, many users emphasized the importance of trialing options prior to purchase and that equipment needed to be more accessible for short-term loan and trialing. One participant reported:

> The only disappointing thing was not being able to trial it for a period before going ahead. Well, where it involved a significant purchase of the equipment, I would prefer to give it a good trial first to see if it would actually work for me and to see if there were any problems.

The time required to trial options varied from a few minutes to months. Some users knew if the device was going to be useful to them immediately, especially if their needs were straightforward or the benefits were immediately obvious, such as reducing glare. One participant told of his experience:

He actually brought a model up to trial for about 1 hour. In that hour, we realized the benefits of having it and so we were making the decision.

Similarly, participants often knew quickly if the device was not suited to their needs. However, when investigating a more complex option, a number of users stated that a 1- to 2-week trial in the work environment was required. One user required some months to evaluate the technology.

Trialing was seen to be important to avoid unnecessary expenditure. One participant noted:

I really need to try things before I buy them because I don't want to spend money and find the damn thing's no better than what I've got.

One participant was able to avoid an unnecessary purchase by trialing the option first and deciding it didn't suit his needs.

Using the technology in the workplace for a period allowed the users to evaluate whether the device was suited to their work environment. One participant noted:

The opportunity to try things out first, very important, preferably in your own environment, though, because the hospital is a very false environment.

One user, whose technology was subsequently found not to work effectively in her work environment, expressed regret at not having an opportunity to trial the option for at least a week prior to purchase.

Trialing was also seen as an important part of exploring the range of options available and determining whether they met the user's specific needs. One participant commented that she found it helpful to trial the range of technologies at the specialist AT service because they could assist her in using devices and discussing the features of each. Trialing also allowed users to evaluate the options available. Another participant had a clear idea what he wanted from a device and evaluated devices against these criteria. In some instances, participants chose not to pursue a technology option after trialing it and discovering its limitations. One participant couldn't imagine having to listen to the voice output of a device for 6 to 8 hours a day. Another found that text enlargement software made it more difficult for him to carry out his work tasks.

In addition to the standard resources for trialing equipment, such as arranging weekly loans from suppliers with loan facilities and on-site trials at specialist services, participants were very resourceful in arranging trialing opportunities. Some trialed options through personal contacts or by locating devices in public facilities, such as a library. A few were able to trial specialist options already available in the workplace, especially in disability-related work environments. However, many week-long trials relied on the goodwill of the supplier loaning the equipment. This often depended on equipment cost and availability. Users reported that the time and costs involved frequently prevented trialing.

In summary, the opportunity to trial a product before making a commitment to it can ultimately save time and resources, as well as help ensure an optimal match of person and technology. Vendors can provide a short-term rental or lease for the purposes of trial periods. By doing so, they will be likely to limit their liability and build rapport with and trust from the consumer.

Keeping Up-to-Date

A number of participants felt it was also important to keep constantly informed about technology developments, either by monitoring technologic developments themselves or by keeping up to date through a technology-literate friend. They reported that this would enable them to find out if there was a new technologic development that might better address their needs. One participant summarized this sentiment in the following statement: *The thing is to keep up with what's available out there and to try it out.*

Keeping abreast of developments also enabled people to identify useful advancements and ensure that they were using the *best* technology and not persisting with outdated equipment. Technologic developments frequently improve the efficiency and comfort for the user, enabling them to work for much longer than they had previously.

Another felt that keeping up with developments enabled him to be better informed about what technology could offer. He commented: If there's no particular need for it at the time, that doesn't mean there's no point in not pursuing it because often, once you accomplish something, you form different ideas on what you can do and gain confidence.

This particular quote also seems to indicate that needs, preferences, and confidence continue to evolve over time and by keeping up, AT users are better able to identify the right product for them at any given point in time.

One participant followed the development of voice recognition technology and waited until laptops developed to a level where they could support the software before purchasing one. He said:

> I saw (voice recognition software) *being used and then starting to look seriously at which laptops it would work on because the quality of the hardware's* (laptop) *very important when using it* (Naturally Speaking).

Employers were also very aware of the need to keep abreast of technologic advances and the implications for the AT user.

Participants used a range of resources to keep up to date with technologic advancements. Although some "kept an eye out," others kept contact with computer-literate friends or read computer magazines, or contacted specialist information services, occupational therapists, or disability organizations. One participant maintained contact with a supplier and checked periodically to see if there had been any useful developments. He reported on a recent experience:

> When I ring her she says "I've been keeping an eye out for you." She knows...I tend to ring people, I have a good talk to them and try to make sure they know your case and that they remember you.

In some workplaces, information technology (IT) personnel also provided the user with information on technology updates that they thought would be helpful to the user and arranged a trial of the devices. For other participants, the Internet provided a way of keeping informed about technology developments.

▨ RECOMMENDATIONS FOR SERVICE PROVIDERS
Technology Possibilities

Being unaware of the technologic possibilities resulted in participants being unable to imagine how technology could assist them. Participants needed to see what technology could do before they could envisage how it could assist them. Those with very little awareness of technology did not seek out possibilities and often encountered a device by accident. Others relied on computer-literate friends to explore options for them and accepted the first option they encountered. Consequently, they were not confident that they were using the best option. It has also been noted that many American AT consumers are only aware of limited alternatives.[40] A number of studies have also found that older people are also only aware of a limited range of assistive devices.[26,30] Even participants who felt they had a good knowledge of computer technology found it difficult to imagine possibilities because of the specialist nature of the technology.

It is important that people with disabilities are able to think freely and to see beyond the external constraints that restrict their vision of what is possible[1] and that they be encouraged to visualize what they want to be able to do so that they can actively explore technologic possibilities.[1] Awareness and knowledge of AT are not only very important to the success of technology solutions, but are also essential to empowering people with disabilities to explore possibilities.[2] To acquire a vision for what is possible, users also need to have contact with other AT users and be exposed to role models who are successfully using AT in the workplace. The more people with disabilities are employed and using technologies effectively in the workplace, the more likely it is that employers, service providers, funding bodies, and people with disabilities will envisage new work opportunities and solutions to job/task restrictions and workplace barriers. Furthermore, service providers need to use an approach designed to involve the consumer in the technology identification and selection process, such as the Matching Person and Technology (MPT) model.[35]

Awareness of Needs

Identifying the right technology requires more than an understanding of technologic possibilities. It also requires an understanding of the person, the functional implications of impairment, the work tasks to be performed, and the environment in which the person is required to perform them. Without a clear understanding of their needs, participants relied on ad hoc methods, trial and error, and suggestions from people they randomly encountered to identify potential options. Of greater concern is that they often persisted with ineffective methods that resulted in discomfort, pain, poor job performance, or potential job loss.

Having a clear understanding of their needs prior to investigating technology options was identified by the participants as essential to the process of identifying the best solution. Furthermore, people must need technology and want it if they are to use it effectively.[36] This is especially important as AT users are often expected to anticipate their technology needs prior to starting a job. Some participants were able to identify their needs independently, whereas others appreciated the assistance of a service provider. In this study, most of the participants with spinal cord injuries felt comfortable with identifying their own needs. It is possible that it is easier to predict the needs of people with impairments that are clearly defined and stable. It has been proposed that people who are uncertain of the functional impact of their disability on task performance may require assistance in identifying their needs.[36] In addition, people with recent injuries may have encountered technologies, other AT users, or professionals who could have assisted them in delineating their needs during hospitalization or rehabilitation. People who are returning to a previous work position would also have a clearer understanding of the demands of the job and the work environment.

AT users with previous limited experience of work or using technology appreciated the assistance of service providers to identify their needs. Service providers were found to be helpful in assisting the user to identify the impact of their impairments on function, setting realistic goals, analyzing tasks, and addressing ergonomic considerations and the demands of current and future tasks and workplace environments. Many service providers have previously recognized the role of service providers in supporting AT users in this way[5,10,22,23,28,39,44]; however, it is heartening that AT users also acknowledged the value of service providers in this role. As noted in Chapter 3, a number of models also highlight that a good technology match requires an understanding of the difficulties employees experience in performing tasks[6,10] and matching the features of the potential devices to the specific needs and skills of the individual, demands of the job and the work environment.[5,10,28,44] In particular, it is important to evaluate the needs of the client within the actual workplace[18,23] and to gain an understanding of the employer's or supervisor's perspective of the job requirements.[23]

AT users want a process that will address all important elements when selecting the most appropriate technology for work. The MPT model and assessment process[35] provide a useful structure that enables the service provider and consumer to work together to identify the most appropriate technology in light of the user's needs and goals, barriers that may exist to optimal technology use, areas to target for training for optimal use, and the type of additional support that may enhance use. It consists of a series of assessment instruments that are organized into three broad areas: (1) determination of the milieu/environment factors influencing use; (2) identification of the consumer's needs and preferences, and (3) description of the functions and features of the most desirable and appropriate technology. Box 4-1 lists the stages of the MPT process and relevant assessment tools.

The Assistive Technology Device Predisposition Assessment (ATDPA)[37] is the measure of most relevance for employees with disabilities selecting a technology to enable them in the workplace. It was designed as a person-centered, ideographic, baseline, and outcomes measure. In a research study of more than 90 vocational rehabilitation counselors and their consumers, the MPT process and assessments were viewed as highly useful.[33]

After the person has received the most appropriate technology for his or her use, the MPT forms may be administered at one or more times after AT acquisition to assess changes in perceived capabilities, subjective quality of life, and psychosocial factors, such as self-esteem, mood, self-determination, and social participation and support. The MPT process is both a personal and collabora-

---

BOX 4-1

The Matching Person and Technology Assessment Process and Instruments

---

The MPT instruments take a personal approach to assessing the potential technology need, choosing the most appropriate technology given the user's needs and goals, the technology features, and environmental support.

Step One: *Initial Worksheet for the Matching Person and Technology (MPT) Model* is used to determine initial goals and potential interventions supportive of goal achievement.

Step Two: *History of Support Use* is discussed to identify supports used in the past, satisfaction with those supports, and those which are desired and needed but not yet available to the consumer.

Step Three: Specific Technology Matching: The consumer is asked to complete his or her version of the appropriate form depending on the type of technology under consideration:

    General: Survey of Technology Use

    Assistive: Assistive Technology Device Predisposition Assessment

    Educational: Educational Technology Device Predisposition Assessment

    Workplace: Workplace Technology Device Predisposition Assessment

    Healthcare: Healthcare Technology Device Predisposition Assessment

Step Four: The consumer and professional discuss factors that may indicate problems with optimal use of the technology.

Step Five: After problem areas have been noted, the professional and consumer work to identify specific intervention strategies and devise an action plan to address the problems.

Step Six: A follow-up assessment is conducted to determine any adjustments or accommodations needed to the technology and to inquire into goal achievement and whether the consumer has changed priorities.

---

tive (user and provider working together) assessment, and the paper-and-pencil measures can also be used as interview guides. As shown in Box 4-1, a range of assessments is offered, from a quick screen, to specialized evaluations (which can be completed in approximately 15 minutes), to a comprehensive assessment (which can be completed in 45 minutes by a trained and experienced service provider). The MPT process is validated for use by persons with disabilities (ages 15 and older), and it is applicable across a variety of users and settings. The measures have been determined to have good reliability and validity, and they have been used in many research studies in North America and Europe. The results of these and other studies show that persons with disabilities report more benefit from and satisfaction with technology as a result of participating in a person-centered process aimed to match them with the most appropriate technologies for their use.

Once the overall goals and role of technology have been determined, the Human Activity/Assistive Technology (HAAT) model[10] provides a valuable framework for defining the specific requirements and specifications of the technology. First, the activities the person is required to perform in the work environment are detailed. It is important to outline the range of activities the person is currently required to perform in the work environment as well as those they are likely to carry out in the near future. Consideration should also be given to how activities performed in other environments, such as the home environment, can also be supported by the technology. Any known programming or storage requirements required by software to perform these activities should also be detailed. Then the current goals and experience of the person are outlined along with their skills and abilities related to the activities and technology. Difficulties they currently experience in performing these activities or using technology should also be noted. The requirements of the workplace environment are then determined by examining existing/proposed technologies with which the device needs to be used, the impact of environment on the technology to be used, the impact of technology on the environment, and the support required by the technology. By tabulating each of the requirements of the activity, person, and environment, it is then possible to detail the specifications required by the technology, as illustrated in Table 4-1.

TABLE 4-1

Defining Technology Specifications Using the HAAT Model

REQUIREMENTS	TECHNOLOGY SPECIFICATIONS
Activity	
Word processing	Input device (keyboard)
Internet searching	Input device (mouse)
Answering phone and taking notes at reception	Additional keyboard or portable system
Photo editing at home	Sensitive mouse option
Person	
Goal to seek advancement in the workplace	Efficient system to maximize productivity
Not confident; limited experience with computers	User-friendly interface
Access speed is slow and effortful	Comfortable keyboard, easily positioned
Repeat errors and mishits evident	Repeat reduction
Familiar with QWERTY keyboard layout	QWERTY keyboard layout
Mouse use awkward	Easy maneuverability and ergonomic position required
Difficulty with double click	Slow double click timing
Difficulty seeing mouse cursor onscreen	Clear screen/pointer magnification
Environment	
Need to work at different workstations throughout day	Portable system
Open plan office	Quiet system
Internet searching, word processing, and photo editing at home	Duplicate system

Once the specifications of the technology have been detailed, it is then possible to search for information about potential solutions and systematically evaluate their capacity to fulfill these requirements.

When identifying the most appropriate device, the quality of professional support also impacts significantly on the outcome for the individual.[31] Service providers need to be very mindful of individual preferences when exploring technology options[45] and the way in which devices contribute to the visibility of disability.[11] Working collaboratively with the AT user is the best way to ensure that the experience and preferences of the user are recognized and considered when identifying the best device.[25,38] Care should also be taken to acknowledge that a particular technologic solution is not the answer for everyone.[34] People should also be informed about simple solutions, offered the opportunity to explore a range of options, and be given the right *not* to choose a technologic solution if that is their preference.[34]

It is also important that workplace accommodations are seen as occurring beyond the point of entry into the workforce. Accommodations need to occur throughout the cycle of employment[14] as responsibilities vary and workplace practices change. As noted in the HAAT model, the dynamic nature of the relationships between the person, the technology, the tasks, and the environment needs to be recognized and the impact of these changes on the user and their AT needs to be addressed.[10] Changes in the individual's needs and skills, the job requirements, and the workplace, as well as developments in computer technology or AT can be addressed through periodic review or follow-up.[10] Similarly, the preferences and attitudes of the employee to AT may change over time, depending on their workplace experiences of success or failure.[45] Although having access to service providers is advantageous, AT users also need to be empowered to be their own *"long-term technologist,"*[17] so that they are equipped to address their changing needs. Rather than seeing themselves as advocates for the employee, service providers should promote "self determination and consumer-directed policies and services" (p. 74)[49] within workplaces so that AT users can take action within the work context to address their ongoing needs. With a sound knowledge of technology possibilities, their needs, and the resources available to them, AT users are better able to navigate the process, set goals, make decisions, and take action.[2]

FINDING OUT

By Accident or through Own Resources

As noted by the participants in this study, some AT users encountered technology by accident. Because of the specialist nature of the technology, it is often difficult for AT users to obtain the information they require. A number of participants expressed frustration with the lack of information available on assistive technology options. This is not unique to this study. These findings are consistent with previous studies in the UK and America, which also reported that access to information on assistive technologies continues to be a problem for potential technology users.[9,12,16] Many AT users and employers continue to struggle to locate resources to provide advice and information on current technologies.[41] Even highly educated people with disabilities have reported that systems providing assistive devices were not clear or readily available to users.[8] AT services have developed rapidly over the last 2 decades, stimulated initially by the availability of new technologies and the passing of antidiscrimination and technology-related legislation. The nature of these services varies considerably from one country to another, and even between regions, owing to legislative differences, the nature of the organizations in which the services were developed, and the availability of resources and personnel. This variation has resulted in a constellation of services being developed that are difficult for consumers to navigate to obtain the information and support they seek; however, the lack of standards for delivering AT services continues to hamper users' access.[16]

A number of the participants investigated technology options independently, and many of them enjoyed this process. Others relied on informal contacts or computer/technology-literate friends to explore options for them. Relying on family and friends for information about assistive technologies has not been found to be as effective as using service providers.[15] Choosing the right device requires both technical knowledge and an understanding of the person's functional capabilities,[22] as well as the demands of the tasks on the environment[10] and personal preferences and characteristics.[34] Selection of the best technology also demands an understanding of the AT user's requirements and preferences, having extensive knowledge of the assistive devices available, their features, and performance tradeoffs.[44] People with a sound understanding of computer technology are not always aware of the limitations of generic technologies in meeting the complex needs of people with disabilities or of developments in the AT industry.

Some participants also commented that exploring options independently required a great deal of time. Although investigating options independently allowed them to develop a broad understanding of the current technologies and services, they often felt that they would have benefited from knowing what they had learned during the process *before* they started. It is clear that having access to people with appropriate expertise can save AT users time and improve their access to information and resources. Some participants also recognized that "being too independent" limited their use of people with appropriate experience. However, some AT users may prefer to rely on informal contacts because they are not familiar enough with technology to ask appropriate questions of people.[12] It has been found that people in less-populated areas where access to professionals is limited are more likely to use this strategy[15]; however, it is also evident that there are other factors at play. People who use this strategy are usually older, have more significant disabilities and lower personal and family income.[15] Working with an informal contact with technology knowledge provides AT users with convenient access to free advice, but this may not result in the user having confidence in the information they receive or the utility of the device.[15]

Some AT users also canvassed suppliers in an effort to find out about the technologies available. Although some found that the information they provided was restricted to the specific devices they sold, others found it useful to maintain ongoing contact with the suppliers in order to track upgrades and new developments.

Service Providers

A number of AT users were either not aware that specialist information resources existed or found out about them during their exploration. This finding is supported by another study that found only 3% to 5% of AT users to be aware of specialist services, despite 7% of them accessing pamphlets and publications from these services.[15] Those who knew about these resources, but did not use them, felt that they should have made better use of them. It has been proposed that many people often do not seek out appropriate agencies or services that could actually have assisted them with technology choices, either because they lack awareness or because of funding complications.[47] It could be that there is a lack of information about these resources or that the services are difficult or costly to access. Alternatively, consumers could be unaware of the processes required to access these resources or may be unclear about the services they offer. As mentioned previously, AT users could also be wary that they do not know enough about technology to ask the right questions.[12]

Many other participants, however, found an independent specialized information service invaluable in providing them with information on potential technologies. With the bewildering array of technologies available, a broad range of people use AT services to assist them in selecting and acquiring technology.[15] It is, therefore, important that centralized information services are adequately funded to ensure that people have access to accurate up-to-date information on the range of technologies available.[16] However, to empower AT users in the long-term, users also need information on the resources available and how to use these effectively to meet their ongoing and changing needs. It is important that users are provided with the information so that they are "informed, demanding and responsible consumers of AT service and devices" (p. 152).[2] Training is also required for service providers to ensure that they are well informed and can provide quality services.[16]

The need to become familiar with the diverse range of technologies available can initially distract service professionals from applying the clinical skills of observation and reasoning that they would readily apply to any other area of intervention. For many professionals, equipment catalogues, fixed and searchable databases, selection hierarchies,[23,45] equipment-based decision trees,[4] and selection matrices[44] provide a concrete way of dealing with their lack of familiarity with devices, the problem of over-choice, and the complexity of the decisions that have to be made. However, these strategies fail to address the specific needs of the individual and the application environment.[43]

Many consider this to be a specialist field that requires knowledge of the range of products and services available and an understanding of how to match people with the "right" technologies.[15] Consumers have called for service providers to have a deeper understanding of how people learn about and obtain devices.[9]

Participants valued information services that provided more than information. Assistance with clarifying needs, device selection, evaluation of the suitability of technology to individual needs, and potential for customization, as well as suggestions for integrating the technology into the application environment may also be provided. Phillips and Zhao proposed that access to supports that assist the consumer with technology decision-making also decreased the likelihood of technology abandonment.[29] Many authors promote the need for formal assessment, especially when users are investigating sophisticated technology options.[5,10,19,22,28,39,44,47]

The support provided to AT users by service providers in rehabilitation services and disability organizations was perceived by participants in this study to be extremely helpful. This support enabled them to locate resources quickly, but also reduced the stress on AT users to locate resources and potential technologies and arrange for trial and delivery. The role of professionals such as therapists and counselors in assisting AT users in the process of identifying the best technology has long been acknowledged in the literature.[20,24,28,32] One survey found more positive attitudes to information and devices among consumers who accessed professionals than those relying on informal contacts.[15] Interestingly, this resource is more likely to be used by people with higher education.[15] As information about technologies becomes even more readily available on the Internet, it is important to acknowledge the value of service providers in assisting AT users to negotiate the complex matrix of information and resources.

Contact with Other Users

In addition to AT services, users also require contact with other AT users to enable them to benefit from the experiences of others and to help ensure that personal choice is maximized.[1,22,38,48] Isolation from AT users made it difficult for the participants to explore the potential benefits and limitations of devices. AT users who did have contact with other users found it useful to discuss devices with people who had experience using them. However, as noted by the participants, their needs often differed from others depending on the nature of their impairment and the demands of work tasks. Although it is a concern for these AT users, isolation from people with similar needs has not been identified previously in the literature. However, having a circle of support that includes people with disabilities has been acknowledged as important by two of the consumer-centered procedural models.[13,22] Although some participants highlighted the benefit of having ongoing contact with other people with similar impairments or using similar technology, there is little in the literature about the advantages of establishing links with other users when exploring technology options. This research indicates that the use of user networks to explore potential technologies requires further exploration.

Internet

The Internet provides consumers with ready access to information, other AT users, and service providers. Increasingly, consumers have easy access to information on technologic developments, as well as the professional literature and research.[8] To ensure that consumers have access to reliable and accurate information, it is important that professionals develop reliable and informative sites. However, not all the information on the Internet can be trusted. It is, therefore, important that AT consumers are well informed about reliable information networks and how and where to access them.[8] In addition, consumers need to understand how to evaluate the credibility and authority of Web sites.

The Internet also provides an opportunity for service providers to be more accessible to consumers. Professionals can detail their services and how to access services on a Web site and can also consult with consumers via an E-mail address. In addition, electronic discussion lists can be developed to enhance communication both between service providers and consumers and within these groups. Models for this type of service delivery are yet to evolve, and funding to support services of this nature is still limited and unpredictable. The information age is changing the professional-consumer relationship. There is potential for the Internet to empower consumers and redress the balance of control in identifying potential AT. For this type of service delivery to be effective, it is essential that consumers and professionals alike be afforded the opportunity to develop appropriate levels of computer literacy and access to computer technology.

Need to Use a Range of Resources

The successful use of AT is dependent on the provision of a broad range of services.[42] AT users felt they benefited from opportunities to talk with an array of people about the technology possibilities. In gathering information from these sources, including independent reading, AT users and their employers felt better able to assess the reliability of information and make more confident choices.

To adequately investigate technology options, a number of questions need to be addressed. Before embarking on the investigation, one must first ask why a device is needed and why one device would be preferable to another. Second, the person needs to determine what devices are available, what they look like, their size, shape, and weight, and what they can do. Next it is necessary to find out where they are available for trial or purchase and the cost of the device from this vendor. In addition, it is useful to know who the device was originally designed for and the persons or tasks to which it is best suited. Finally, the user needs to know how to use it; adjust it to meet individual needs; and how to service it, troubleshoot problems, or fix it if it stops working. A range of information resources are available to AT users and service providers, each of which contributes to a solid understanding of the technologies available and their suitability.

Suppliers and company catalogues are resources that are readily accessed and answer the *what* and *where* questions. That is, they provide clear graphics and detailed specifications of devices and provide an accurate price and a list of suppliers. Many assume that a device is required, promoting devices within their range, and rarely explore nontechnologic options. Generally, information on who the device was designed for or is best suited to is readily available; however, the vendor is not typically in a position to determine if the device suits the specific needs of the individual or to customize the device to the unique requirements of the individual. Suppliers are often well placed to provide an overview of the features of devices and, in some cases, can provide support in how to use it. In addition, a reliable supplier also will be available for servicing and repairs. To make good use of a supplier or company catalogue, the consumer or service provider needs to have a clear understanding of the specific requirements the person has of the technology. In addition, it is helpful to have an understanding of the full range of options available and how this specific range compares with other options of other vendors. It is also useful to access people with some experience in using the devices or with knowledge about how well the devices meet the needs of a range of users.

Databases also provide users and service providers with information about what devices are available and where they can be purchased. Although databases generally provide information on a broad range of devices, unless they are managed and updated regularly, information on prices and availability can sometimes be out of date and restricted to the country or region that manages the database. Whether graphics and detailed specifications are provided varies depending on the database. However, databases frequently describe the features of devices using key labels, which enable the consumer to compare easily the specifications of devices within a range. Search functions also enable the user to search for specific features, but the sophistication of this function varies from one database to another. Once again, databases automatically assume a device is the logical answer to the question being posed. Similar to suppliers and catalogues, effective use of a database relies on first having a clear understanding of the person's specific requirements and what is expected of a device. In addition, contact with people using the options being investigated and knowledge of how well the devices meet the needs of a range of users are invaluable in making effective use of the information gained from this resource.

Specialist AT information services also often have managed databases, which are available directly to the consumer or are accessed by the service provider in response to a consumer query or need. These services provide comprehensive and unbiased information on the full range of AT devices. In addition to providing the benefits of databases already outlined, these services also have providers who can assist the consumer in determining if they require a device and then in identifying the features most suited to the individual's specific requirements. In addition, the service provider can undertake an advanced search or call on their clinical experience to identify the range of devices best suited to the consumer. The AT service provider would generally have an understanding of who the device was designed for and how well it might meet the needs of a range of people. Depending on his or her experience, an AT service provider also may be able to adjust it to the user's specific requirements and instruct the user in fundamental aspects of device use. However, the AT service provider may not have sufficient experience in using the device on a day-to-day basis to support the user in troubleshooting problems that might arise. The service provider also should be able to direct the user to information on maintenance and servicing. This information resource is well suited to people who do not have a great deal of experience in identifying their needs or using technology. The service provider can assist the individual in clarifying goals and needs and exploring options other than devices. They also generally have experience with using the devices with a range of people, and they understand the strengths and limitations of devices. In addition, they have an understanding of the local suppliers and the quality of after-sales support available as well as local trialing and training facilities. Because they regularly access the literature on product development and application of technologies, they also are generally well informed about technologies on the horizon and issues requiring consideration in the selection and application of technologies.

Talking with other AT users helps people with disabilities benefit from the experiences of others in selecting and using devices. It allows them to discuss and clarify issues, such as what devices are in use, how well they work and the quality of local after-sales support and servicing. AT users who have day-to-day experience with using devices in a number of applications are able to discuss compatibility issues and share shortcuts and troubleshooting strategies. AT users groups generally have members who track technologic developments and discuss the potential suitability of these to their specific needs.

INDIVIDUAL APPROACHES TO THE PROCESS

It is clear that people have very different levels of interest in exploring technology, and that this diversity of knowledge and interest needs to be recognized in the nature of resources and support provided for AT users. Although some AT users require direct access to information systems and resources, others appreciate the assistance of service providers in identifying their needs and locating potential options and appropriate resources. AT users with an active interest in exploring technology require access to diverse information sources. These users make good use of information systems and require easy access to catalogues, product reviews, and databases. Managed AT databases that are regularly updated and manned by professionals also provide consumers with access to experienced professionals who are available to clarify needs and assist the AT user in understanding the range of technologies and resources available.

AT users with a limited interest in technology and knowledge of resources require service providers to actively inform them of the broad range of technologic possibilities and promote the available services. This can be achieved by providing information leaflets or case examples to illustrate the potential of technology and by accessing consumers directly through newsletters and support groups. Additionally, specialist AT professionals can provide indirect support to consumers by educating employment and health service providers through advertisements and articles in professional newsletters, in-services, or workshops, and by presenting at relevant conferences. Managed information systems are also a valuable resource for service providers supporting AT users through this process. These information systems are regularly updated and manned by professionals who can assist people in identifying their technology needs as well as understanding the range of technologies available. Service providers and AT users benefit from these services, through which they can be informed of recent technologic developments and be helped in locating relevant resources.

To date the heterogeneity of AT users has not been adequately addressed in the literature. Although many service providers assume the AT user is reliant on their professional advice,[3,46] some consumer advocates propose that AT users prefer to be completely self-reliant.[17,47] This research has shown that AT users sit at various points along this continuum, and that service providers need to develop a range of approaches and resources to meet their various requirements. Being aware of the heterogeneity of AT users enables service providers to be more responsive to the diverse needs of consumers. Consumer-directed services are also more likely to result if a range of consumers is involved in the development and operation of these resources. Appendix A provides comsumers with questions to guide their exploration of technology options and direct their use of resources.

▪ TRIALING

The participants in this research stressed the importance of trialing equipment prior to purchase to avoid unnecessary purchases. They felt that there were three benefits to trialing equipment. First, it allowed the user to explore a range of options. Second, the user was able to determine whether he or she felt comfortable with the device. Third, it provided the user with an opportunity to evaluate his or her suitability in terms of accommodating his or her impairments and meeting the job demands as well as ability to operate within the work environment.

Because the time required for trialing devices ranges from a few minutes for simple devices to weeks for complex devices, a range of resources need to be made available. Where possible, AT users have arranged weekly loans from suppliers, some of whom had loan facilities or through onsite trials at specialist services. However, these trials frequently relied on the goodwill of the supplier loaning the equipment and depended on equipment cost and availability. AT users also arranged trials through personal contacts and locating devices in public facilities, such as a library. Occasionally, they were able to access specialist options already existing in the workplace. However, many felt that the time and costs involved in trialing equipment prevented them from benefiting from this valuable experience.

The value of onsite trials has been acknowledged in the literature,[18,22] especially trials over an extended period, for example, 2 to 5 days.[18] It is likely that discomfort may not be experienced over a few hours, when trialing equipment in a show room; however, it may be evident following several days of use. Extended onsite trials can also prevent abandonment, as obstacles to optimal use can be identified and addressed prior to purchase.[40] It has been proposed that it is more effective if the user learns to use the device prior to trialing,[6,7] so that the user has the required skills to use the device safely and effectively. In instances in which this is not possible, support needs to be provided to assist the user in operating the device. It is also important that the device is fitted and adjusted to optimize the effectiveness of the trial.[6] Questions designed to guide the user to make good use of a trial are provided in Appendix B.

▨ KEEPING UP WITH TECHNOLOGIC DEVELOPMENTS

Participants felt that keeping up with technologic developments enabled them to identify useful advancements and ensure that they were using the best technology. They used a range of resources, including reading computer magazines, contact with computer-literate friends, specialist information services, occupational therapists, or disability organizations. Only a few participants indicated that they actively used the Internet to keep up with information on technologies. Similarly, a recent survey of AT users found less than 1% of respondents using the Internet.[15] This system could be underused because people with disabilities have limited access to computer technology and the Internet. A recent report indicated that only 33% of people with disabilities in America (compared with 56% for able-bodied people)[27] had access to computer technology and only 16% had Internet access at home (compared with 34% for able-bodied people).[21,27] In addition, they could be unskilled in locating appropriate resources on the Internet. It is also difficult to evaluate the quality of Internet-based information without some knowledge of the equipment and confidence in the reliability of the site. The information also may be overwhelming to people who have limited experience with technology. In addition, people may need more assistance in identifying their needs and exploring a range of low- and high-tech options rather than relying solely on the product-oriented databases currently available.

When outlining best practice principles, Angelo et al. urged service providers to remain current with technologic developments to match accurately the appropriate technology to the client's needs.[3] With the rapid development of technology, it is also essential that the technology user be provided with independent information about potential technology developments. The AT user and service providers need to access people with the right expertise to assist them in understanding the new developments and their potential for people with disabilities. Specialist AT information services provide a valuable service. Their databases are managed by specialist professionals, ensuring that people receive reliable, quality information and have access to a qualified professional.

Many authors in the United States have called for improved access to this information.[6,7] In the UK, Cowan and Turner-Smith further advocated that "resource centres, local information services and support groups should be known to and promoted by all professionals involved in the rehabilitation process" (p. 5).[12] Furthermore Andrich and Besio argued that awareness and knowledge of AT are essential to empowering people with disabilities and ensuring the success of the devices.[2] To this end they have provided a user-centered educational model that informs users about information resources, the range of technologies available, as well as issues related to the selection, acceptance, and utilization of these technologies. This educational approach aims to empower users to improve their quality of life by informing them about the technologic possibilities. In addition, it seeks to develop their capacity to select AT not only by providing information on devices, resources, and service systems but also by discussing issues that are likely to affect their choices.[2]

SUMMARY

This chapter has detailed the experiences of AT users in identifying the right technology in this first step of the process of choosing and integrating technology into the workplace. Knowing what was technologically possible and being aware of their needs formed a critical foundation to this step. AT users used various sources to find out what was available, ranging from encountering options accidentally or through their own contacts to using formal mechanisms. Although the Internet has become an important source of information, users acknowledged the need to access a broad range of information sources. It is also apparent that users vary in their interest and understanding of technology, and that this should be reflected in the range of resources made available to them. Of particular interest to all users is the opportunity to trial devices. Trialing allows individuals to explore the range of options and to determine whether the device is comfortable to use and adequately meets their requirements. Keeping abreast of the developing technologies is a challenge for the AT user and service provider alike. The Internet is an information source that has the potential to both inform and overwhelm. Its power as a medium for service delivery is yet to be harnessed and provides an ongoing challenge to service providers and AT users to use it effectively for information exchange and support.

References

1. Alliance for Technology Access: *Computer and Web Resources for People with Disabilities.* Berkeley, Calif, Hunter House, 2000.
2. Andrich R, Besio S: Being informed, demanding and responsible consumers of assistive technology: an educational issue. *Disabil Rehabil* 24(1-3):152-159, 2002.
3. Angelo J, Buning ME, Schmeler M, et al: Identifying best practice in occupational therapy assistive technology evaluation: an analysis of three focus groups. *Am J Occup Ther* 51(10):916-920, 1997.
4. Anson DK: *Alternative Computer Access: A Guide to Selection.* Philadelphia, FA Davis, 1997.
5. Bain BK, Leger D: *Assistive Technology: An Interdisciplinary Approach.* New York, Churchill Livingstone, 1997.
6. Bazinet G: Assistive technology, in Karan OC, Greenspan S (eds): *Community Rehabilitation Services for People with Disabilities.* Boston, Butterworth-Heinemann, 1995.
7. Behrman MM: Assistive technology training, in Flippo KF, Inge KJ, Barcus JM (eds): *Assistive Technology: A Resource for School, Work and Community.* Baltimore, Paul H. Brookes, 1995.
8. Brooks NA: Models for understanding rehabilitation and assistive technology, in Gray DB, Quatrano LA, Lieberman ML (eds): *Designing and Using Assistive Technology: The Human Perspective.* Baltimore, Paul H. Brookes, 1998.
9. Brooks NA: Users' responses to assistive devices for physical disability. *Social Sci Med* 32(12):1417-1424, 1991.
10. Cook A, Hussey S: *Assistive Technologies: Principles and Practice,* ed 2. St. Louis, Mosby, 2002.
11. Covington GA: Cultural and environmental barriers to assistive technology, in Gray DB, Quatrano LA, Lieberman ML (eds): *Designing and Using Assistive Technology: The Human Perspective.* Baltimore, Paul H. Brookes, 1998.

12. Cowan D, Turner-Smith A: The user's perspective on the provision of electronic assistive technology: equipped for life? *Br J Occup Ther* 62(1):2-6, 1999.

13. Dailey P, Scherer M.J: Mobilizing my resources, in Alliance for Technology Access (ed): *Computer Resources for People with Disabilities: A Guide to Assistive Technologies, Tools and Resources for People of All Ages,* ed 4. Alameda, Calif., Hunter House Inc., 2004.

14. Dowler DL, Hirsh AE, Kittle RD, et al: Outcomes of reasonable accommodations in the workplace. *Technol Disabil* 5:345-354, 1996.

15. Ehrlich NJ, Carlson D, Bailey N: Sources of information about how to obtain assistive technology: findings from a national survey of persons with disabilities. *Assistive Technol* 15:28-38, 2003.

16. Galvin JC: Assistive technology: federal policy and practice since 1982. *Technol Disabil* 6:3-15, 1997.

17. Gradel K: Customer service: what is its place in assistive technology and employment services? *Vocational Rehabil* April:41-54, 1991.

18. Hammel JM, Symons J: Evaluating for reasonable accommodation: a team approach. *J Prevention Assessment Rehabil* 3(4):12-21, 1993.

19. Hawley MS, O'Neill P, Webb LH, et al: A provision framework and data logging tool to aid the prescription of electronic assistive technology. *Technol Disabil* 14:43-52, 2002.

20. Inge KJ, Wehman P, Strobel W, et al: Supported employment and assistive technology for persons with spinal cord injury: three illustrations of successful work supports. *J Vocational Rehabil* 10:141-152, 1998.

21. Kay H: *Computer and Internet Use among People with Disabilities.* Washington, DC, National Institute on Disability and Rehabilitation Research, 2000.

22. Kelker K, Holt R: *Family Guide to Assistive Technology.* Cambridge, Mass, Brookline Books, 2000.

23. Langton AJ, Ramseur H: Enhancing employment outcomes through job accommodation and assistive technology resources and services. *J Vocational Rehabil* 16:27-37, 2001.

24. Lash M, Licenziato V: Career transitions for people with severe physical disabilities: integrating technology and psychosocial skills and accommodations. *Work* 5:85-98, 1995.

25. Law M: *Client-Centered Occupational Therapy.* Thorofare, NJ, SLACK Inc., 1998.

26. Mann WC, Tomita M, Packard S, et al: The need for information on assistive devices by older persons. *Assistive Technol* 6:134-139, 1994.

27. McKinley W, Tewksbury MA, Sitter P, et al: Assistive technology and computer adaptations for individuals with spinal cord injury. *Neuro Rehabil* 19:141-146, 2004.

28. Nochajski SM, Oddo CR: Technology in the workplace, in Mann WC, Lane JP (eds): *Assistive Technology for People with Disabilities,* ed 2. Bethesda, MD, AOTA, 1995.

29. Phillips B, Zhao H: Predictors of assistive technology abandonment. *Assistive Technol* 5:36-45, 1993.

30. Roelands M, Van Oost P, Buysse A, et al: Awareness among community-dwelling elderly of assistive devices for mobility and self-care and attitudes towards their use. *Social Sci Med* 54:1141-1451, 2002.

31. Rogers JC, Holm MB: Assistive technology device use in patients with rheumatic disease: a literature review. *Am J Occup Ther* 46(2):120-127, 1992.

32. Rumrill PD, Garnette M: Career adjustment via reasonable accommodations: the effects of an employee-empowerment intervention for people with disabilities. *J Prevention Assessment Rehabil* 9:57-64, 1997.

33. Scherer MJ: Assessing the benefits of assistive technologies for activities and participation. *Rehabil Psychol* 50(2):132-141, 2005.

34. Scherer MJ: *Living in a State of Stuck: How Assistive Technology Impacts the Lives of People with Disabilities,* ed 2. Cambridge, Mass., Brookline Books, 1993.

35. Scherer MJ: *Living in a State of Stuck: How Assistive Technology Impacts the Lives of People with Disabilities,* ed 3. Cambridge, Mass., Brookline Books, 2000.

36. Scherer MJ: The impact of assistive technology on the lives of people with disabilities, in Gray DB, Quatrano LA, Lieberman ML (eds): *Designing and Using Assistive Technology: The Human Perspective.* Baltimore, Paul H. Brookes, 1998.

37. Scherer MJ: *The Matching Person & Technology (MPT) Model Manual and Assessment,* ed 5, [CD-ROM]. Webster, NY, The Institute for Matching Person & Technology, Inc., 2005.

38. Scherer MJ, Craddock G: Matching Person & Technology (MPT) assessment process. *Technol Disabil* 14:125-131, 2002.

39. Scherer MJ, Galvin JC: An outcomes perspective to quality pathways to the most appropriate technology, in Galvin JC, Scherer M (eds): *Evaluating, Selecting, and Using Appropriate Assistive Technology.* Gaithersburg, Mass., Aspen, 1996.

40. Scherer MJ, Vitaliti LT: Functional approach to technological factors and their assessment in rehabilitation, in Dittmar SS, Gresham GE (eds): *Functional Assessment and Outcome Measures for the Health Rehabilitation Professional.* Gaithersburg, MD, Aspen, 1997.

41. Sidoti C: *The DDA and Employment of People with a Disability,* 1998. Retrieved October 10, 2004, from www.hreoc.gov.au//disability_rights/speeches/1998/employment_98.html.

42. Smith RO: Measuring the outcomes of assistive technology: challenge and innovation. *Assistive Technol* 8:71-81, 1996.

43. Sowers JA: Employment for persons with physical disabilities and related technology. *Vocational Rehabil* 3:55-64, 1991.

44. Sprigle S, Abdelhamied A: The relationship between ability measures and assistive technology selection, design and use, in Gray DB, Quatrano LA, Lieberman ML (eds): *Designing and Using Assistive Technology: The Human Perspective.* Baltimore, Paul H. Brookes, 1998.

45. Struck M: Technology solutions for ADA compliance. *Occup Ther Health Care* 11(4):23-28, 1999.

46. Trefler E (ed): *Assistive Technology.* Thorofare, NJ, Slack, 1997.

47. Turner E, Barrett C, Cutshall A, et al: The user's perspective of assistive technology, in Flippo KF, Inge KJ, Barcus JM (eds): *Assistive Technology: A Resource for School, Work and Community.* Baltimore, Paul H. Brookes, 1995.

48. Turner E, Wehman P, Wallace JF, et al: Overcoming obstacles to community re-entry for persons with spinal cord injury: assistive technology, ADA and self advocacy. *J Prevention Assessment Rehabil* 9:171-186, 1997.

49. Wallace JF, Gilson BB: Disabled and non-disabled: allied together to change the system. *J Prevention Assessment Rehabil* 9:73-80, 1997.

Acquiring Technology for Work

■ "My AT has meant the difference between me not being able to work and to work."—AT Study Participant

A lthough knowing that enabling technologies are available reassures people with disabilities, gaining and sustaining employment is dependent on being able to acquire the "right" technologies. In Chapter 5 the second stage of the process of selecting and using technology in the workplace is considered (Figure 5-1). In the first part of this chapter, the experiences of assistive technology (AT) users in acquiring their technology are described, whereas the second part of the chapter provides recommendations for service providers based on the AT users' experiences of this stage of the process. This chapter aims to address the issues encountered by AT users during this stage including: (1) retaining control over decisions, (2) the amount of time taken to obtain the technologies, (3) the expense of the technology and associated costs, (4) accessing adequate funding, (5) the flexibility of the funding, and (6) additional and ongoing costs.

■ USER EXPERIENCES

Although some AT users need only low-tech solutions, such as typing splints, mouthsticks, or wrist supports, or add-ons such as alternative keyboards (Figure 5-2), tracker balls, and enlarged monitors, others require specialized software such as text enlargers, screen reading, and voice recognition software or specialized equipment such as closed circuit television and Brailler. The details of the types of technology used by participants who contributed to this study can be found in Table 5-1. The cost of these technologies ranged from a few hundred to thousands of dollars.

Control over Decisions

Some users had limited control over decisions regarding the work-related technologies they acquired. For example, a number had personal contacts that independently identified a need and provided a solution to the user, frequently without being asked and often without consulting the user. Mostly these people were well intentioned. One participant recalls his experience:

I don't remember ever formally saying can you do this, or him saying I'll do it, but I remember him saying yeah you know I'm working on something and bingo it's there.

Similarly, there were AT users who had access to rehabilitation professionals who were engaged by their employer to identify suitable AT for their work situation. After an initial consultation with the user, the professionals sometimes

111

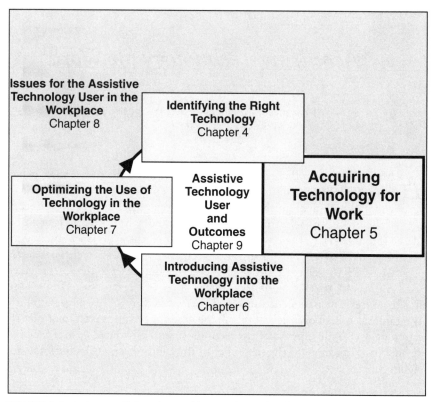

FIGURE 5-1 ■ Stages of choosing and integrating technology into the workplace.

gave their recommendations directly to the employer, who arranged the purchase of equipment without involving the user in further discussion. Some participants accepted this approach:

It was basically on her (the professional's) *recommendation. I think that she was the expert in that field. She knew of different things. She looked at me, I suppose, and looked at my position, work situation, and decided that would have been the one that best suited me. And me with my temperament, I've just gone along with it. It has worked well.*

One user expressed her frustration that professionals assumed control for decision-making. She recalled that she had to actively regain control during the selection of her technology option, saying: *There were these two* (rehabilitation professionals) *who had their own ideas but I forcibly got what I wanted....But it wasn't what they wanted.*

On reflection one participant lamented that he had been dissuaded from buying a laptop by the funding body and instead had bought a less expensive desktop. He regretted not dealing directly with the insurance company and getting the laptop he wanted. He noted:

You have to be very assertive, particularly if you are dealing with an insurance company, because they tend to push things on you. At the time I really wanted to get that

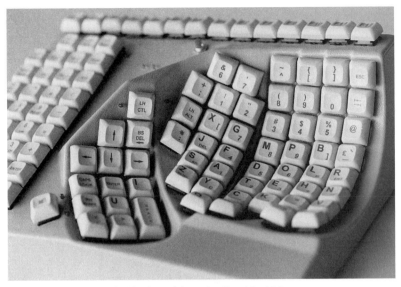

FIGURE 5-2 ■ One-handed keyboard (Royalty-Free/Corbis).

laptop computer so that I could be more mobile and they said: "No, you don't want a laptop, get a PC." I said: "No. I really want a laptop." In the end I was basically cornered into getting the PC and I found that was the worst decision. I should have got the laptop. So, I wasn't assertive enough at that stage to do that. I know a lot more now.

AT users who were involved in the decision-making process considered that their involvement was critical to the success of the outcome. This allowed them to express their preferences and to extend the service provider's understanding of their needs beyond the existing job as illustrated by this exchange:

Researcher: *So you had a fair amount of determination about what technology you purchased.*

Participant: *We had to find out what was necessary for this position but also what would be necessary if I moved on. What we ended up getting would be beneficial to me if I decided to find other work.*

Additionally, technology changes in the workplace can also significantly affect decisions about the type of technologies available to AT users. One participant reported that he was being encouraged to change over to another voice recognition program because the workplace was upgrading their technology and moving to a particular platform. He was reluctant to change brands because it would require relearning and retraining. He was also uncertain of the reliability of the new brand. After some discussion, his employer agreed to go with his preferred option. The participant explained:

The department is moving to a new corporate desktop and so (the voice recognition software) has to be upgraded. The department is going to be moving to (another brand). They'll be reluctant to support (my product) because of the arrangements

Text continued on p. 118.

TABLE 5-1

Assistive Technologies Used by Participants

INITIALS	DIAGNOSES	FUNCTIONAL IMPAIRMENT	WORK TASKS PERFORMED BY PARTICIPANTS	ASSISTIVE TECHNOLOGY USED
A	C5-6 spinal injury	Mobility: manual wheelchair	Word processing PowerPoint	Typing splints Trackball
B	Rheumatoid arthritis	Mobility: electric wheelchair Manipulation: adaptations	Word processing E-mail/web Telephoning	Compact keyboard/voice recognition Graphic tablet mouse Hands-free phone
C	C4-5 spinal injury	Mobility: electric wheelchair	Word processing E-mail/web telephoning	Naturally Speaking Marble Trackball Hands-free
D	Spinal muscular atrophy	Mobility: electric wheelchair Manipulation: mouthstick	Word Processing/spreadsheet -Email/web Telephoning	Onscreen keyboard Hands-free
E	Amputation arm/shoulder	Manipulating two-handed tasks	Word processing Telephoning Driving	Compact keyboard Headset for phone Adaptations
F	Spinal injury from birth	Mobility: electric wheelchair	Word processing telephoning	Access Pack Head set
G	Vision impairment from birth	Severe short-sightedness	Reading and writing Data entry and management Microfiche	Closed-circuit TV Text enlarger Enlarged screen
H	Overuse syndrome	Decreased manipulation	Word processing Desktop publishing, database entry	Voice recognition Trackball

TABLE 5-1

(cont'd)

INITIALS	DIAGNOSES	FUNCTIONAL IMPAIRMENT	WORK TASKS PERFORMED BY PARTICIPANTS	ASSISTIVE TECHNOLOGY USED
I	C4-5 spinal injury	Mobility: electric wheelchair Manipulation: mouth/ headstick	Data entry telephoning	Access Software, Keywiz, headpointer, macros Phone with headset Tried voice recognition
J	Cerebral palsy	Mobility: walks with limp Manipulation	Word processing and Excel Desktop publishing and power point E-mail Phone	Hands-free phone
K	C4-5 spinal injury	Mobility: electric wheelchair Manipulation: typing sticks	Word processing Spreadsheets E-mail/telephone	Voice recognition Typing sticks Trackball Mounted handset
L	Acquired vision impairment (1985)	Vision: peripheral shadows	Reading Word processing E-mail/web	Kurzweil Personal Reader Screen reader Text enlarger
M	Cerebral palsy	Mobility: electric wheelchair Manipulation: head pointer Communication: difficult to understand	Word processing Telephoning	Headpointer Hands-free
N	C3 spinal injury	Mobility: electric wheelchair Manipulation: support staff	Text entry E-mail/web telephone	Voice recognition Trackball Mouthstick Hands-free

TABLE 5-1
(cont'd)

INITIALS	DIAGNOSES	FUNCTIONAL IMPAIRMENT	WORK TASKS PERFORMED BY PARTICIPANTS	ASSISTIVE TECHNOLOGY USED
O	Cerebral palsy	Mobility: electric wheelchair Manipulation: uses straw to drink Communication: dysarthric	Windows 95 Invoicing program	Keyguard Joystick mouse
P	Cerebral palsy	Mild mobility impairment Mild manipulation impairment	Spreadsheets Word processing Telephoning	Wrist supports Word prediction, Access software Standard telephone
Q	C5-6 spinal injury	Mobility: electric wheelchair	Accounting package Phone	Typing splint Access Pack Omnikey Ultra Dragon Dictate(start)
R	Multiple sclerosis	Mobility: electric wheelchair Manipulation: severely affected	Accounting package MYOB Word processing Web and e-mail Phone	Naturally Speaking Through computer
S	Vision impairment	Severe short-sightedness	Data entry Word processing/spreadsheet Desktop publishing/e-mail	Closed-circuit TV Zoomtext
T	Vision impairment	Vision: total loss of vision	Reading Word processing, Excel/ E-mail/web Notetaking Listening to taped manuals/docs Message taker/item and doc marker	Brailler/scanner/tape recorder Screen reader Braillite business memo device Perkins Brailler

TABLE 5-1

(cont'd)

INITIALS	DIAGNOSES	FUNCTIONAL IMPAIRMENT	WORK TASKS PERFORMED BY PARTICIPANTS	ASSISTIVE TECHNOLOGY USED
U	C5-6 spinal injury	Mobility: manual wheelchair Manipulation: finger splints	Text entry Telephoning	Finger splints Trackball/arrow keys Hands-free
V	C4-5 spinal injury	Mobility: electric wheelchair mouthstick	Word processing Phone	Voice recognition
W	Multiple sclerosis	Mobility: electric scooter	Text input/telephone Filing/photocopying	Standard computer/telephone Scooter
X	C4 spinal injury	Mobility: electric wheelchair	AutoCAD Word processing Desktop Publishing Scanner OCR	Typing splints Modified Trackball Naturally Speaking Hands-free phone
Y	C2 spinal injury	Mobility: electric wheelchair Manipulation: support staff Breathing: ventilator	Word processing/e-mail telephoning	Dragon Dictate 2.52 Headmaster mouse Hands-free
Z	C4-5 spinal injury	Mobility: electric wheelchair	Word processing Phone	Typing splints Mobile phone Voice recognition

they've got. So they asked me to have a look at transferring over to (the new product), which I had a look at their package and I'm not at all happy with it, so I'm looking at upgrades (for my software).

This case illustrates the importance of the user being actively included in decision-making regarding workplace changes and needing to be assertive when new technologies are being acquired. The previous cases show the value consumers place on being a part of the decision-making around technology selection and how crucial their involvement can be to productive use.

Time Taken to Obtain Technology

Participants reported that delays in the supply and installation of technology were a significant barrier to using technology in the workplace. Virtually all participants experienced considerable delays in acquiring their technology. One participant recalled:

The people that supplied (the device) *were supposed to supply it with a remote system. That arrived about 12 months after I actually had the device and they won't fit it for me.*

Many participants identified delays in obtaining the required technology as an issue they would like addressed.

Some participants reported that they regretted that they were not more proactive in requesting assistance. One commented:

I think I would have done things a lot quicker but it's a bit hard when you're just starting your job; you don't want to make too many waves. I think battling constant headaches and eyestrain is not a particularly good idea just to hold down your job. So probably I should have done things earlier than I did.

One employer also was disappointed in the time it took for the employee to get around to looking at technology options. She said:

The time that was taken, was the time (the employee) *got around to going and having a look and, you know, that was the most significant time and that may have taken a few months.*

The participants proposed many other reasons for delays in acquiring the ideal technology, such as the workplace using outdated technology, having limited access to computers, delays in the approval process for funding, and supplier delays. Some participants were limited in their technology options because the workplace had not yet established an infrastructure for using technology or did not have adequate computer facilities for the employees. One participant noted: *To a large extent, we're still working the old way. The computers are still a bit of a treat.* Frequently participants had to wait for computer equipment to be upgraded in the workplace before their technology could be purchased and installed. Platform upgrades were often tied to main budget expenditures in the workplace, and employers were unaware of the impact of these delays on the user's work performance. Similarly, orders for expensive specialized technologies were also tied to larger workplace IT orders, which were contracted out, and dependent on tenders. Delays of 12 months for the processing of these orders were not uncommon.

After these upgrades were completed, the user often had to wait further for their specialized technology to arrive. Some participants were disappointed in the delays in acquiring devices from the supplier. They were aware of the limitations in supplying specialized equipment, as suppliers frequently had limited stock owing to the cost and limited turnover of the equipment. Often this equipment had to be imported, which caused further delays.

Participants commented that because of the original funding agreement, they had to arrange for new equipment to be purchased when changing jobs. One technology user, who was in the process of changing employment, commented that a quick turnaround time was essential in enabling her to move into her new position and maintain her continuity of employment. Another user, who had recently moved into a new position, was fortunate in being able to pass information about his technology requirements to the IT department in his new workplace, who arranged for the equipment to be installed and ready for use when he commenced work.

Expense of the Technology

Specialized and customized computer technology can be very expensive. Although voice recognition technology has become cheaper over the years, the more reliable brands cost more than $1,000 at the time these participants acquired their technology. This technology also required a powerful computer to run effectively, further adding to the cost of the system. For participants who were working for themselves or in a small company, these additional costs prevented them from buying the AT they needed.

> *At the moment, I'm just using normal products. I've been considering for a long time the possibility of purchasing a software program that you can dictate to, Voice Recognition software. The thing that has restricted me there is cost at this stage. Not so much the software itself; it's just that I would like it on my laptop. My laptop is too small for the requirements of the software. I've decided I can't outlay the money to purchase that at this stage.*

The costs alone often prevented the AT users, especially those on disability pensions, from exploring technology possibilities. Others who were on a modest salary self-funded their work-related technology up to $10,000. One participant stated:

> *It was all self-funded, so I had to borrow some money and I was hoping to offset some of the cost with the sale of my old Braille display and the scanner or reading machine that I have at home, as well as the stand-alone reader, but I've had a lot of trouble trying to sell those so I'm still in debt.*

One employer highlighted the discrepancy between the cost of mainstream technology and the cost of equipment for people with disabilities in the following comment:

> *I just wish there were something that could be done about the pricing of these* (specialized technologies). *I know there's a lot of work that goes into this sort of equipment, but I can go and buy a mouse for $14.00.* (The AT User) *has to go and buy one for nearly $900.00—you know it's a lot more costly for him.*

Many AT users were also responsible for self-funding their home technologies. This cost was often additional to what they had already invested in equipment for work. One participant lamented the need for a headpiece at home as well as work.

Some participants reported that they could never afford to fund their personal computer needs at home because of the cost of the specialized technologies and felt that funding should be made available for these purchases as well. One participant stated:

Anything that helps you in this instance has got to be seen as essential to living and life so I think they should be funded.

Participants also felt a need to keep up with the latest technology and update their systems regularly to be competitive with their able-bodied peers. One participant commented:

You do need to update and if you're going to compete with people who have all their physical attributes, then you need cutting edge technology. See you can't walk away from it. It's just a pity that cutting-edge technology is so expensive.

Again, the cost of regularly updating their technology was prohibitive for many.

Accessing Adequate Funding

Participants in this study received funding from a range of sources for their work-related technologies. Six participants purchased technology entirely from their own funds, and one bought his equipment with money from a third-party insurance claim. Twelve participants received funding through a nationally funded government rehabilitation service, with two augmenting this with their own funds. Seven participants received funding from their employers to purchase their technology, with two also contributing some of their own funds toward the purchase of devices.

A number of the participants felt that the technology was so essential to enabling them to perform their work tasks that they were prepared to purchase the technology themselves if they were not able to secure adequate funding. One participant commented:

If the Department didn't fund (the device), *would I fund it myself?...Categorically, totally, yes, I would.*

Participants who were self-employed generally purchased their own technology. One participant felt that the cost of this technology limited his options:

It's a bit difficult funding it all yourself...I will have to go cheapskate if I can't find any help with any employment options.

Many participants who received initial assistance (government, community funds, or worker's compensation) to purchase equipment felt that this initial funding was essential to their employment. A number of employers, however, were unaware that government funding was available.

Many participants commented that they had to be very persistent to secure funding; it required them to explore a range of funding programs or write to their local government representative. One participant commented on the persistence she required to secure her funding:

I knew I would have gone right down to the very last, to my local Member at that time. You know you still might have ended up with "no," but that was the worst you could get, isn't it.

In addition, of those who received initial funding, few were confident they could secure such funding again. One reported: *I don't think anybody else will ever get one like I got this. I'm sort of the last one. I just got in under the wire so I don't think that's sort of being done again.* Many had to purchase subsequent equipment and upgrades themselves.

When government funding was secured, participants reported that their choices were constrained by a ceiling of $5,000. One participant expressed his dissatisfaction with this limit, reporting that an additional $1,000 for the split screen Closed Circuit Television (CCTV) would have increased his efficiency enormously.

In those instances in which the employer funded equipment, participants and their employers reported that money for equipment (and upgrades) was often taken out of their work budgets. One employer described this:

> *That'll probably cost us a few thousand dollars from what I can see, but I mean that's not very much really, in an organization of this size. I'm putting the hard word on our workplace people to provide it, but it will probably end up coming up out of our budget.*

One participant limited his request because the costs of the equipment came out of his budget, as illustrated in this discussion:

> *I got the employer to agree to buy me a new computer next year. So I don't think I can, you know, say "look, give me another $400 for a program"... if I asked and they'd give it to me but they'll probably take it out of my budget.*

Knowing that their technology was affecting the budget of their department or organization often caused concern to the AT user, particularly those who worked in small businesses and community organizations with restricted budgets.

Flexibility in Funding

For some participants the equipment was funded for their individual use, which enabled them to take the technology with them when they moved to another place of employment. These users continued to make good use of these technologies in their new jobs and appreciated the flexibility that this provided them. Another user who was establishing his own business received a loan from a rehabilitation service to purchase his equipment and then repaid the loan over time. This enabled him to acquire the equipment he needed to establish his business.

Additional Costs and Ongoing Costs

It was reported that AT also resulted in additional costs for the employer in terms of upgrading platforms, the time and training required to learn to use the new technology, and the cost of IT support to keep the technology operational. Two participants reported that their employers declined their requests for AT because of the cost that would be incurred by the employer in upgrading the existing computer technology platform or providing a standalone computer that would not be fully utilized. Although funding for specialized technology was available, one participant was unable to utilize this because the employer was not willing to upgrade the existing work platform. One participant reported that the employer was concerned also about the down time required for the user to become proficient in using the new assistive technology and the cost of having equipment that was being underutilized because it had been customized to the needs of a specific individual. He said:

> They were looking at the costings and everything else within their budgets and about how much down time was required on the equipment, that was a major problem particularly when it wasn't networked, or even if it was networked, and the amount of available resources on that machine.

In addition to meeting the ongoing costs of upgrading technology, participants also reported that funding needed to be extended to cover IT support and training. These are often overlooked when technology needs are being costed, but are especially important considerations for people who work in small businesses and organizations or in regional areas without access to IT resources or ongoing funding. The frustration of one employer regarding these additional funding requirements is summarized in this quote:

> Limited financial resources is definitely an issue and within this region, the actual training of the program and having someone on hand who has skill or experience with it was very severely lacking.

Where IT support was available through the workplace, some participants appeared to be well supported with relatively standard technologies. Not all participants had access to this type of support. One participant found that he had to limit his technology choices because of the lack of technical support available within the workplace. However, many participants sought the assistance of people informally to provide the IT support they required. Frequently these services were provided as a favor or at reduced cost.

Participants reported that they needed to change their assistive technology after 2 to 4 years because of changes in their functional ability, failure or unreliability of the old technology, upgrading of workplace platform or software, or because there had been developments in technology that provided them with more effective options. The employer or the AT user generally met these ongoing costs themselves. However, frequently, the AT users continued to use outdated, inadequate technology or ineffective methods to carry out their work tasks. One participant elaborated on the need for ongoing funding in the following quote:

> It would be useful to have funds available, particularly since it's pretty necessary. Once you're in employment there have been big changes with computers. What was adequate for me 4 years ago isn't now.

One well-informed participant was very aware of his ongoing needs and the resultant costs that he bore in keeping his technology up-to-date, so he made sure that the cost of upgrades was included in the initial purchase cost. He stated:

> Work doesn't cover any (upgrading) costs. I'm involved with that. The latest upgrade was a free one because we bought a software maintenance agreement with the previous major update. And I think it does make the suppliers more ready and willing to offer support, too, when you've got that you pay that little bit of extra and have that agreement.

A coworker nominated by one of the participants was also a service provider who supported the AT user in acquiring his AT in the workplace. This was an example of a work environment with a high level of integration, where AT users were supported by skilled people within the organization. She acknowledged the need for appropriate training, especially when using sophisticated technology such as voice recognition. She applied for funding for training in the original submission for AT. She noted:

> *I think that's one thing that people really need to be very much aware of before they go in and purchase it. We had to do that as part of the submission that we wrote, to get funding for the equipment* (and for training as well).

Training was so important to one participant that she paid for it herself and hoped that her employer would reimburse her.

▓ RECOMMENDATIONS FOR SERVICE PROVIDERS

Although the quotes, examples, and cases provided are from technology users in Australia, all of the issues discussed occur just as frequently in Europe and the United States in spite of legislation such as the Americans with Disabilities Act. Thus, the issues and discussion that follows apply globally.

Control over Decisions

For some users, an acquaintance or a professional took control of decisions regarding their technology. Some AT users were grateful for the assistance of a third party, whereas others resented the control being taken from them. They did not feel their needs were being adequately met as they were not able to evaluate the potential of devices in meeting their current or future requirements. In addition, AT users who are not actively involved in the process are not offered the opportunity to become aware of the range of options and resources available to them. Consequently they are then reliant on others to address their future technology needs.

The importance of involving the user in decision-making regarding technology has been highlighted repeatedly in the literature.[2,4,5,13,22,28] It is not only critical in reducing device abandonment,[23] but also is an essential part of client-centered practice.[13] It was evident in this research that AT users varied in their level of interest in technology and that this affected the time and attention they were prepared to allocate to understanding their technology. However, to manage their long-term technology needs, consumers are encouraged to develop an awareness of the resources available, the range of options in the market, and an understanding of the features that will assist them with their work tasks. This will enable them to be actively involved in decision-making and equip them to better address their future technology needs. Service providers need to be sensitive to the AT user's level of interest and understanding of technology, ensuring that they allow novice users to direct the process without overwhelming them with information and responsibilities. When working with these AT users, service providers need to ensure that they do not automatically assume responsibility for the process and the decisions that are made along the way. On the other hand, AT users with an active interest in technology often require access to a range of resources and expertise. These users need to actively direct the decision-making process and should not have to assert themselves to be heard by the service providers. Collaborative approaches such as proposed by the MPT model[25] can assist service providers and AT users in working together to gain an understanding of each other's perspective and determining the best solution.

Comments from AT users reinforce the importance of actively involving them in choosing and acquiring their technology. AT users' personal preferences, as well as their long-term needs, must be taken into consideration when making decisions about technology. This not only reduces abandonment,[23] it also ensures good use of the technology in the short and long term. Appendix C provides a series of questions to assist AT users in choosing the best technology for their needs. It is also imperative that the employer and employee are actively involved in the process. This facilitates the immediate success of the intervention[27] and provides both parties with an understanding of the process and the resources available to meet their ongoing needs.

Time Taken to Obtain the Technology

AT users find the delays in acquiring technology for work problematic. Consistent with the experiences of the participants in this study, timely acquisition and delivery of technology has been found to be a problem by other AT users.[3,7,11] This research identified a number of reasons for delays in acquiring technology. Delays resulting from importing equipment from overseas were expected. However, there were additional unexpected reasons for delays. Some AT users were initially slow to act on the difficulties they were experiencing in the workplace, perhaps out of concern for seeming to be too assertive or demanding. AT users need assurance that their technology requirements are legitimate and require clear, supportive processes for addressing these. They also benefit from information on how technology can assist them in their work tasks and need ready access to resources to assist them in identifying suitable options. Delays also resulted from slow approval processes in the workplace or having to wait for current computer platforms to be upgraded. Employers need to be made more aware of the urgency in meeting the AT users' technology needs and the need to separate these orders from main budget items. Service providers also need to work with employers and IT personnel to ensure that workplace platforms and technologies are upgraded quickly to support AT users' technology needs. Workplaces with limited or outdated technologies present barriers to people with disabilities. Service providers also should be working with employers to identify technologies that accommodate the AT user's impairment and also enable them and other employees to work more efficiently. Delays in acquiring appropriate technologies limit AT users' productivity in their current workplace and reduce their mobility within the workforce and, hence, their career path. AT users are not able to respond to new employment opportunities if processes for addressing their technology needs result in long delays.

Expense of the Technology

Although many mainstream technologies continue to decrease in price, AT tends to maintain their high costs. The expense of these specialized technologies remains a major obstacle for people with disabilities,[3,7,20,30] especially those who are self-employed or on pensions. Although the Job Accommodation Network (JAN) reported that most accommodation costs were less than $1000 in 1995, it is often difficult to determine the actual costs of workplace accommodations.[17] Accommodations for people with more significant disabilities who require sophisticated technology can be in excess of $10,000 to $15,000.[17,21] These costs are often compounded by having to purchase a more powerful computer to support their specialized technology. In addition, people with disabilities need to regularly upgrade their technology to stay competitive in the workforce. These ancillary costs have not been identified in the literature to date and need to be acknowledged if funding bodies and AT service providers are to meet the "real" needs of AT users. Furthermore, whereas the cost of technology in the workplace has predominated in the discussion, little is known about how AT users fund their technology needs at home. Some AT users in this study reported that they had to fund a duplicate of their workplace technologies for home use. Unfortunately not all AT users can manage this expense.

Research shows that people with disabilities are not accessing computer technology and the Internet to the same extent as the rest of the community.[16,21] It might be easy to assume that this is because they have specialized technology needs; however, there is a growing realization that it is a social rather than a technologic issue. Without suitable technologies in the home, people with disabilities are becoming increasingly excluded from interactive digital communications, resulting in a "digital divide" between those who can afford computer technologies and those who cannot.[12] This lack of access means that people with disabilities are not able to make use of the very resources that would give them access to the information that can enable them to participate in the community.

Accessing Adequate Funding

AT users emphasized the importance of being able to access funding to assist with the purchase of specialized technologies. Funding through government rehabilitation schemes has been available for some time; however, it is of concern that some employers remain unaware of them. In addition, it is clear that AT users who were successfully employed had to be persistent to access this funding and remain doubtful of accessing further funding. Lack of adequate funding has been widely reported as a major obstacle to the acquisition of appropriate technologies.[2,7,30] Because there are few established funding sources for assistive technologies, AT users have to be imaginative and assertive to access and utilize funding effectively, often procuring money from a range of sources to cover their expenses.[1] It is no surprise that potential technology users often abandon the search for funding because of the complexity and uncertainty of the funding programs.[28] It is, therefore, important that employers and AT users be fully informed about the financing options available to them and that processes are streamlined so that they can be readily accessed. Service providers can be very helpful in assisting AT users in identifying potential funding sources and systematically exploring their funding options[17]; however, it is also important that AT users develop a funding strategy to meet both their immediate and long-term technology needs.[1]

Many AT users accessed funding from government rehabilitation schemes or their employer. Although this funding enables them to purchase essential devices, a number of AT users also supplemented this with their own funds to meet all their technology needs. It is understandable that government funding programs have needed to cap costs by setting a limit for expenditure, but basing considerations on costs alone should be avoided.[17] For some AT users the allocated budget is more than they require, and employees are often encouraged to spend the remaining funds on additional devices. In other cases, however, this ceiling limits the options available to the AT user and means that he or she has to settle for a less-than-adequate solution or supplement the cost out of pocket. Accommodations need to be determined based on a thorough review of the employee's specific needs and circumstances,[17] rather than working to a specified budget. Funding bodies need to develop better strategies for evaluating the requirements and priorities of each individual to ensure that money is allocated wisely. Routine evaluation of the outcomes of AT accommodations will provide funding bodies with information on the effectiveness of the accommodations they fund and assist them in developing a structure for decision-making that will enable them to prioritize purchases that compete for limited funding.

Complexities arise that require careful consideration when employers are responsible for accommodations. First, if employers are uncertain about what is required to facilitate the productivity of a person with a disability in the workplace, it can make employing a person with a disability a complex proposition. In their study of outcomes following accommodations in the workplace, Dowler et al. reported that employers were initially fearful of the costs involved in accommodations, but subsequently reported cost benefits in terms of hiring and retraining, increased productivity, prevention of future injuries, and avoiding litigation.[9] The challenge is to provide employers with adequate information and support so that they are able to address the AT users' accommodation requirements and recognize the potential benefits of employing a person with a disability. Second, whereas the antidiscrimination legislation addresses large employers, many AT users are employed in small businesses and community organizations where the financial resources for accommodations are limited. This means that the AT user's' technology requirements often place a burden on the budget of these workplaces. They are acutely aware of this fact. They may be reluctant to request what is needed and opt to finance their requirements from their personal budgets. Finally, once an employer purchases the required technologies and undertakes the necessary upgrades to the workplace to enable them to operate effectively, it is difficult for the AT user to move within the workplace or to another organization because the equipment stays with the employer.[1] Initiatives such as cooperative agreements, in which the costs of accommodations are shared between the employer and vocational rehabilitation schemes, help allocate costs and delineate ownership between the government and workplace. However, these could be extended to provide AT users with assurances regarding their rights to equipment.[17]

Flexibility in Funding

Some authors have cautioned against funding programs in which the AT user is dependent on others to fund expensive technologies, because this results in AT users accepting an option that they would not otherwise choose[20] or perhaps feeling tied to that place of employment. To ensure AT users have independence and mobility in the workforce, alternative funding strategies need to be explored. With independent funding options, AT users can purchase their preferred technology and move into new positions and change jobs without having to renegotiate their equipment needs with each successive employer. Independent funding sources such as loan schemes[29] afford AT users greater autonomy as they are able to take equipment with them when they relocate or change employment. Since not-for-profit loan financing programs were first established for assistive technologies in the United States, they have continued to flourish.[30] These programs provide flexible loan terms with below-market interest rates to assist people with disabilities in meeting their technology requirements. AT users have taken loans ranging from $500 to $20,000 to purchase computers and adaptive software, as well as vehicles, vehicle modifications, home modifications, and hearing aids.[30] Because people's AT needs are rarely confined to one context,[10] these loans also enable AT users to meet their needs across application environments (both work and home).

Tax advantages for AT users and employers have also been proposed to reduce the financial burden of AT to individuals and employers. In the United States, AT users receiving such benefits as Social Security Disability Insurance (SSDI) or Supplementary Security Income (SSI) are able to deduct some of their AT expenses from their additional earnings to retain their benefit status.[1,21,29] In addition, careful documentation and timing of expenditures can relieve much of the cost of impairment-related work expenses and accommodations for individuals and businesses.[1,29] Although these tax incentives have proved useful for employers in covering the costs of accommodations,[17] equipment purchased by AT users using federal tax incentives under the Americans with Disabilities Act remains the property of the employee,[15] thus affording them flexibility of future employment. However, little is known about how often these self-directed funding options are used and for what purposes they are most appropriate.[14]

Additional and Ongoing Costs

Financing AT is considered to be the most significant problem faced by individuals with disabilities in the workplace[22,26] and a major barrier to successful employment.[11] However, in addition to the costs of the technologies, there are other costs that have not been acknowledged to date in the literature. The costs of upgrading existing platforms, addressing network incompatibilities, and supporting specialized technologies are an ongoing drain on workplace budgets. In addition, the costs of down time for skill development and having dedicated equipment being underutilized are a concern for employers. Without an understanding of these costs, unrealistic expectations will continue to be made of employers, who not only meet the initial cost of the specialized technology but also cover the incidental costs incurred. It is important to understand employers' needs, priorities, and perspectives to support their commitment to employing people using AT in the workplace.[18] When extensive accommodations are required, it has been proposed that the responsibilities of funding bodies and employers be clearly delineated through contracts that designate ownership, liability, and provisions for the repair and maintenance of the technologies.[15] This is particularly important for small businesses and community organizations, where many AT users find employment. These employers are often unable to meet these expenses or experience difficulties in meeting the needs of employees with specific requirements. Although businesses with less than 20 employees are exempt from providing accommodations under the unjustifiable hardship clause,[19] they are reluctant to leave employees with disabilities without the technology they require to perform their job effectively. Large organizations are better able to cover these additional costs, whereas smaller organizations would benefit from tax incentives to reduce the stress these costs place on workplace budgets.[11]

Consideration also needs to be given to the ongoing needs of the AT user. It is well recognized that computer technology has a limited lifespan[24]; however, no funding provisions currently address the ongoing costs of technology. Funding also needs to cover a range of technology support services such as evaluation, training, repair/maintenance, and upgrading of equipment.[22] AT users found it very helpful when funds were allocated for training, IT support, and subsequent upgrades in the initial purchase package. However, this funding must often rely on service providers estimating the future needs of the AT user prior to purchase,[6] rather than being available to the user as required. Maintenance is also important if equipment is to be used to its full potential and, therefore, this needs to be included in funding packages.[7] Funding needs to be available to AT users who work in small businesses and community organizations, who are often unable to bear these additional costs. If governments are not in the position to provide access to ongoing funding, policies similar to those developed in the United States[11] that allow tax sheltering for acquiring, maintaining, and upgrading expensive technologies would reduce these financial burdens.

Currently, funding schemes are primarily focused on acquiring work technologies to facilitate or maintain employment.[29] Although these address AT users' immediate technology needs, they do not meet their ongoing technology requirements. Workplace accommodations need to be viewed as an ongoing expense rather than a one-time purchase. For many participants, funding was only provided when they started a new job or when they were at risk of losing their job. This meant that they were not readily able to change or upgrade their technology when their function or work tasks changed, the technology became outdated or unreliable, or workplace computer systems were upgraded. The constant evolution of technology also means that developments and improvements can significantly improve the outcomes for people using AT. However, they are often unable to take advantage of advances in technology, because they are costly or the current systems have insufficient speed or memory to accommodate an updated technology. Extending the financial support over a number of years, as is the case in the UK, with approved costs being covered over a 3-year period,[8] comes some way toward recognizing the ongoing costs associated with using AT in the workplace.

Service providers need to be aware of the limitations of the current funding systems and optimize AT users' access to these. They also need to actively advocate for systems that meet the demand more realistically. Funding bodies require a better understanding of the real costs and repeated expenses that AT users incur and the implications of placing these costs on the employer. Although one-time funding grants for equipment help meet the needs of AT users, a deeper understanding of their ongoing needs is required if AT users are to remain productive in the workforce. AT users also need information on funding sources to address their ongoing needs. Questions are provided in Appendix D to guide AT users in acquiring and funding their technology.

This study investigated AT users who were successful in acquiring and maintaining employment. A greater understanding of AT users who struggle to acquire appropriate technologies or who are forced to persist with ineffective options is required if funds are to be allocated equitably and funding systems that meet the true needs of the AT user and their employer are to be devised.

SUMMARY

This chapter examined the experiences of AT users when using their technology at work. Although AT users appreciate assistance throughout the process, they value being actively involved in decision-making, as this enables them to understand the range of options available and the strengths and limitations of these. It also affords them with opportunities to explain their requirements and preferences, and better equips them to deal with their ongoing needs. The experiences of AT users in this second stage of the process have also highlighted that timely recognition of need, as well as acquisition and delivery of technology, are critical to the viability of AT users in the workforce. Additional costs, such as evaluation, training, IT support, repair and maintenance, and subsequent upgrades, also need to be recognized and suitable mechanisms for addressing these expenses established. Funding systems also need to be more flexible to ensure that AT users are not tied to one place of employment and can access the full range of employment opportunities. Alternative funding schemes, such as loans, tax incentives, and leasing arrangements should be investigated further to determine their potential for providing AT users with greater autonomy and flexibility. This research has also highlighted the precarious position of many AT users in terms of funding their ongoing technology expenses.

Greater involvement of consumers in the development of funding systems would also assist in developing more consumer-responsive funding options.

References

1. Alliance for Technology Access: *Computer and Web Resources for People with Disabilities.* Berkeley, Calif., Hunter House, 2000.
2. Bain BK, Block L, Strehlow A: Survey report on the assessment of individuals with spinal cord injuries for assistive technology. *Technol Disabil* 5:289-294, 1996.

3. Booth M: *Access and Compatibility Issues: A Survey of Consumers.* Paper presented at the Australian conference on technology for people with disabilities, Adelaide, South Australia, October 9-12, 1995.

4. Butterworth J, Kiernan WE: Access to employment for all individuals: legislative, systems and service delivery issues, in Lehr DH, Brown F (eds): *People with Disabilities Who Challenge the System.* Baltimore, Paul H. Brookes, 1996.

5. Cook A: *Assistive Technology Trends in North America.* Paper presented at the Third Australian Conference on Technology for People with Disabilities, Adelaide, November 25-28, 1997.

6. Cook A, Hussey S: *Assistive Technologies: Principles and Practice,* ed 2. St. Louis, Mosby, 2002.

7. Cowan D, Turner-Smith A: The user's perspective on the provision of electronic assistive technology: equipped for life? *Br J Occup Ther* 62(1):2-6, 1999.

8. Curtis J: Employment and disability in the United Kingdom: an outline of recent legislative and policy changes. *Work* 20:45-51, 2003.

9. Dowler DL, Hirsh AE, Kittle RD, et al: Outcomes of reasonable accommodations in the workplace. *Technol Disabil* 5:345-354, 1996.

10. Enders A: *Technology for Life in a New Disability Paradigm.* Keynote presentation at the Fourth Australian Conference on Technology for People with Disabilities, Sydney, September 28-30, 1999.

11. Galvin JC: Assistive technology: federal policy and practice since 1982. *Technol Disabil* 6:3-15, 1997.

12. Goggin G, Newall C: *Digital Disability: The Social Construction of Disability in New Media.* Lanham, Md, Rowman & Littlefield, 2003.

13. Gradel K: Customer service: what is its place in assistive technology and employment services? *Vocational Rehabil* April:41-54, 1991.

14. Hagner D, Cooney B: Building employer capacity to support employees with severe disabilities in the workplace. *Work* 21:77-82, 2003.

15. Hammel JM, Symons J: Evaluating for reasonable accommodation: a team approach. *J Prevention Assessment Rehabil* 3(4):12-21, 1993.

16. Kay H: *Computer and Internet Use among People with Disabilities.* Washington, DC, 2000, National Institute on Disability and Rehabilitation Research.

17. Langton AJ, Ramseur H: Enhancing employment outcomes through job accommodation and assistive technology resources and services. *J Vocational Rehabil* 16:27-37, 2001.

18. Lash M, Licenziato V: Career transitions for people with severe physical disabilities: integrating technology and psychosocial skills and accommodations. *Work* 5:85-98, 1995.

19. Lunt N, Thornton P: Country policy reports: Australia. *Employment Policies for Disabled People: A Review of Legislation and Services in Fifteen Countries.* York, Social Policy Research Unit, University of York, 1993.

20. Lupton D, Seymour W: Technology, selfhood and physical disability. *Soc Sci Med* 50:1851-1862, 2000.

21. Mc Kinley W, Tewksbury MA, Sitter P, et al: Assistive technology and computer adaptations for individuals with spinal cord injury. *Neuro Rehabil* 19:141-146, 2004.

22. O'Day BL, Corcoran PJ: Assistive technology: problems and policy alternatives. *Arch Phys Med Rehabil* 75:1165-1169, 1994.

23. Phillips B, Zhao H: Predictors of assistive technology abandonment. *Assistive Technol* 5:36-45, 1993.

24. Rohl JS: *Technology Directions and Their Impact on the Way We Work*, 1998. Retrieved September, 2000, from *www.doplar.wa.gov.au/w&f/wfcr/rohl.html*.

25. Scherer MJ: *Living in a State of Stuck: How Technology Impacts the Lives of People with Disabilities*, ed 4. Cambridge, Mass., Brookline Books, 2005.

26. Sowers JA: Employment for persons with physical disabilities and related technology. *Vocational Rehabil* 3:55-64, 1991.

27. Steinfeld E, Angelo J: Adaptive work placement: a "horizontal" model. *Technol Disabil* 1(4):1-10, 1992.

28. Turner E, Barrett C, Cutshall A, et al: The user's perspective of assistive technology, in Flippo KF, Inge KJ, Barcus JM (eds): *Assistive Technology: A Resource for School, Work and Community*. Baltimore, Paul H. Brookes, 1995.

29. Wallace JF: Creative financing of assistive technology, in Flippo KF, Inge KJ, Barcus JM, eds: *Assistive Technology: A Resource for School, Work and Community*. Baltimore, Paul H. Brookes, 1995.

30. Wallace JF, Hayes M, Bailey MN: Assistive technology loan financing: a status of program impact and consumer satisfaction. *Technol Disabil* 13:17-22, 2000.

CHAPTER 6

Introducing Assistive Technology into the Workplace

■ "(Before getting my new AT) I relied on other people constantly…I would say it probably took on average (in terms of) paid time of people, about 30% of their productivity time, which meant our productivity was down."—AT Study Participant

Once the user has purchased the technology, it is vital that it is set up properly in the workplace to enable them to function independently. When the device is delivered, the user embarks on the third stage of the process, *introducing the technology into the workplace* (Figure 6-1). In this stage of the process, assistive technology (AT) users are faced with the complexities of setting the technology up so they can use it to carry out their work tasks without disruption to their own productivity or that of their peers. Frequently the user is reliant on a number of devices, which need to be set up and integrated with generic equipment in the workplace.

This chapter first explores AT users' experiences of using technology in the workplace and the strategies and supports that assist them in making their technology operational. It then examines how service providers can promote the productivity and inclusion of AT users in the workplace. This chapter examines the following issues AT users experience when introducing their technology into the workplace: (1) the reliability of the technology, (2) accessing technical support, and (3) operating as efficiently and as effectively (as others) in the workplace environment.

■ USER EXPERIENCES
Reliability of the Technology

AT users reported having ongoing compatibility problems with a variety of software and commented on the many hours volunteered by friends and acquaintances to try to resolve these difficulties. One AT user told of her reliance on her friend to resolve a compatibility problem:

I used to try to run sticky keys with AutoCAD and that used to always kill it, and my friend spent lots and lots of time trying to sort that out, so again if I did not have him…well, I would not have made it.

Without these informal supports, some AT users had to learn to resolve these difficulties on their own. One AT user commented: *it's sink or swim…you've got to learn…to find out yourself.* It was evident that a number of AT users were

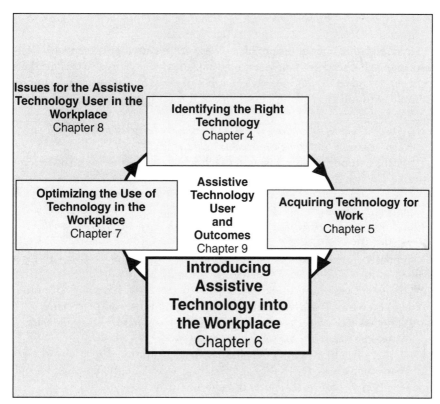

FIGURE 6-1 ▪ Stages of choosing and integrating technology into the workplace.

dealing with similar difficulties and were not aware that other people were also trying to resolve the same issues. The examples provided in this chapter illustrate both resourceful resolutions and frustration when an acceptable solution is not found.

Some resourceful users contacted the supplier to try and resolve compatibility problems. However, they often experienced ongoing difficulties despite continued contact. In some cases, the software developers were aware of the problems and had plans to resolve them in future upgrades of the software. This provided little comfort for the AT user in the workplace.

Furthermore, the AT users were often using cutting edge technologies or combinations of technologies that had not yet undergone field testing. As a result, users discovered difficulties before the developer was even aware of them. One employer supporting a contract worker commented on the delays experienced in getting cutting edge technology to work:

It's OK to access all this equipment, but it would have been better if we were able to have someone there to help us set it up rather than finding out it's not working, talking over the telephone, then sending it back and waiting another month or 6 weeks or so before you can access that equipment again.

In addition to encountering difficulties with technology incompatibilities, users found that some of their technology was unreliable. This also became more apparent as the technology aged. A number of people using voice recognition technology found that changes in their voice resulting from illness or fatigue decreased accuracy. One AT user noted:

If I have a cold or if I'm tired, it fails—it's not nearly as good; so therefore it just exacerbates your frustration when you're tired anyway.

Another stopped using his aging technology altogether when it became unstable. He stated:

(The voice recognition program) wouldn't work at all on my computer. It kept crashing out all the time. We de-installed it, then re-installed it, re-trained it and it'd work, and we go back the next day to use it and crash, it'd just jam up and wouldn't work at all.

Similarly, mainstream software or hardware upgrades in the workplace resulted in the AT user experiencing difficulties. In some workplaces upgrades occurred every 2 years. One user expressed his frustration with having to readdress problems each time there were technology changes in the workplace. He said:

Every time they change computers or programs, this [program] starts to muck around, and you have to play with it and get it to work.

AT users felt that many of the issues they encountered in the workplace could have been averted with forward planning. One AT user expressed his opinion when his system crashed after it had been upgraded:

They (the workplace) knew that the computers were going to be changed and certain new software was going to be added on. I suppose a forward-thinking person could just do that trialing with the software. They could have perhaps taken (the software) and stuck it on a computer and played with that and it certainly would have solved a lot of problems. Just to trial it beforehand and then solve the problems before they got here.

At times, functions in an existing system were no longer available to the AT user in the updated software. In particular, the change to Windows technology had a significant impact on people with disabilities. It resulted in a number of the AT users having to investigate an effective mouse alternative:

I only needed the keyboard at that stage. Then I came here I needed the mouse, and I think that was another reason that I was finding it a bit of a problem too.

Some users reported that having a backup system for their AT was useful when their main technology was not operational, that is, when their computer was down or their AT was being repaired. One AT user spoke about the value of having a high- and low-tech backup:

I have two electric wheelchairs because I won't rely on one. Technology can have its failures too and because I'm so reliant on technology, you've got to have back up, and these typing sticks are my backups for (voice recognition software).

Having an alternative or backup system also provided AT users with more flexibility in terms of how they carried out their work tasks. One AT user appreciated being able to alternate between technologies as shown in the following comment:

If I don't feel like talking for (voice recognition software), *I will type; and just say one day I've got a really sore elbow and I can't be bothered typing, I use* (voice recognition software).

One well-informed user who worked in a technologically proficient workplace spoke of the benefits of using computers with removable hard drives. He proposed that having a removable hard drive with all his software loaded would allow him to quickly reinstall his special software on another computer if his system crashed.

Accessing Technical Support

AT users expressed a need for ongoing IT support within the workplace. Those who work in workplaces without IT personnel used a number of strategies to address their needs. As noted previously, some relied on "superusers" in the workplace or IT-literate friends. Others learned about the technology themselves so they knew how to deal with recurring problems. However, a number of users purchased specialist support that was costly to either themselves or their employer. For many, the cost of this support was prohibitive, especially to AT users who were self-employed. One user protested:

I'm spending more than half my money on just keeping this damn thing afloat. It costs arms and legs. If that damn thing crashes, I have to pay for it.

AT users experienced difficulties getting adequate support even for mainstream software, such as voice recognition software. As their *only* means of text input, program management, and cursor control, people with disabilities rely on this technology more extensively than their nondisabled counterparts and frequently use it in combination with other specialized and mainstream technologies. Mainstream suppliers and IT personnel often did not understand the nature of the difficulties they were experiencing or the urgency of the problem.

Poor product support also meant that there were often long delays in addressing problems or in obtaining repairs and maintenance. Even in workplaces with good IT support there were delays when dealing with companies servicing specialized equipment. These delays had a significant impact on productivity. One AT user commented:

Yes, getting it fixed is sometimes a problem, especially finding a person in the area that can repair these types of machines. Last time it broke down...it took about four weeks or so to get it fixed, so that was a bit of a problem.

Not surprisingly, employers expressed concerns and frustration with the slow response time for repairs and maintenance of their employees' technology. One employer stated:

We have had difficulties with the maintenance people in that they promise a 3-day turnaround and, in fact, despite my calls, it was quite a difficult situation for the employee and for us, because he was having to cope with that (without his essential technology).

However, some AT users found the manufacturers and suppliers to be very responsive to their questions and requests for adjustments to their products. Although improvements were not always immediately available to the AT user, they appreciated suppliers who provided ongoing after-sales services to their clients. Having access to people who really understood the software was invaluable as illustrated in this quote:

The fellow who came out from the supplier was an absolute guru in the software, so if we had a hiccup, he knew exactly what to say, how to do, where to fix it.

One AT user felt that purchasing the hardware and software from the same supplier improved one's chances of getting backup support. He stated:

If you go to a hardware specialist and get your hardware and then go to a software specialist and get your software, if something goes wrong, you send it back to the software people, they say oh no, it's a hardware problem; if you go to the hardware people, they say it's a software problem. You need to get an integrated package from one area.

Employers also valued support from the suppliers. One employer recalled:

The technology was not compatible with (the desktop) *program. We had difficulty in that everything would function OK with a standard mouse, but once we plugged the joystick in it was different. We sent the joystick back and they worked on it and resolved it for us.*

Having ready access to technical support with experience in the installation and maintenance of specialized technologies was seen to be essential by AT users. For some users, the IT personnel in the workplace provided ongoing support for maintenance and compatibility issues as reflected in this statement: *The IT division installed the software and then gave sort of any support for it.* In some large government departments, the human resource personnel took responsibility for addressing technology problems experienced by employees with a disability. One AT user expressed his satisfaction with this system in the following quote: *I usually report the matter to the HR section and they organize for a repairer to fix it.* The quality of support received from IT personnel depended on the skill of the person who attended to the problem, as illustrated in this quote:

We've got computer people, like in the call center; they did all the basic stuff. Anything more involved and it really falls down to one or two guys at the computer center. There's one guy in particular who was involved a lot with the OT when it was first set up and he knew a few subtleties about it to make it work.

One user emphasized the importance of having access to the right expertise when he said:

Researcher: So that was useful to have that resource (specialist) *there to ensure that your technology was operational for you.*

Participant: Essential, totally essential...having him there, to sort out the software problems, meant the difference between going and not going because our people, that is our technical people, just didn't have the knowledge or know-how or the understanding of (the software), *to be able to work it.*

Operating as Efficiently and Effectively in the Workplace

AT users sometimes experience difficulties using their technology because of the nature of the workplace environment. For example, people using voice recognition technology often experienced difficulties in open office environments. Noises in the environment resulted in inaccuracies or system crashes—in one case up to three times a day. One AT user abandoned the technology because she was not able to use it effectively in her workplace. Another AT user was also conscious of the distraction she might be causing her coworkers in using the voice recognition technology. Other technologies were also a problem in shared workspaces. One AT user with vision impairment tried to restrict his use of a Braille printer because of the noise it created. This AT user's employer stated:

> The noise of some of the equipment is annoying. See, the Braille printer must be about "5,000 decibels" and it's most frustrating, but it needs to be convenient for the employee. I suppose we just have to put up with it, at the moment because we haven't yet got the money to buy a proper cover (for the printer).

In some workplaces, AT users shared workstations with coworkers. This meant that the user had to rely on their coworkers' ability to understand their specific requirements, so that they could disengage and reset the special technology for the AT user when they left the workstation. This was particularly an issue for AT users who worked part-time. Where some AT users found the coworker to be obliging in this regard, others found coworkers were unable to understand their requirements, despite their best intentions. One AT user was unable to access the computers at work because they were a shared resource and were placed on desks that were not accessible for him.

AT users also were unable to move around the workplace environment as their colleagues did. They commented that, although their coworkers often worked at other workstations, they were locked into a specific workstation with their AT. This meant that if they were required to work at another workstation, they experienced discomfort, strain, or decreased work performance. One AT user illustrated his restrictions in this quote:

> If I need to use someone else's workstation, I have to go back to my old ways because they don't have (specialized software).

Consequently, many AT users felt that a laptop offered them much more flexibility than a desktop computer in enabling them to move about the workplace and to use their technology in a range of environments. One AT user commented:

> I really like the laptop...that really suits my needs because I can pack it up and push it away and I don't have to look at it all the time. It's not confronting me like a big wall like a desktop, so I'm happy with that.

Having a laptop also enabled some AT users to continue to work at home, for example when they were ill. One AT user recalled:

> If I ended up in bed for a period of time, as has happened to me in the past, I can just put the laptop there by the bed on the trolley and use it.

In addition, having a removable drive enabled one user to take his software with him when working at other workstations or locations.

Furthermore, having an AT system that offers a range of input or output modes provides the user with flexibility when undertaking a variety of tasks, in a range of environments. One AT user commented:

> And what I really like with this one (specialized product) is the fact that it has the option to turn the speech off. Sometimes I get so sick of listening to synthetic voices

with the earphones on and having to concentrate on a voice, but having just the Braille display for a lot of stuff I need to read and study. It's much better to have the detail of the Braille and it's something I can just read quietly, take notes quietly, and check things back in a meeting or in a taxi or wherever I am, which is, I think, far less antisocial than clattering away on a Braille machine or having to rely on putting a headphone on and listening to speech all the time.

Most AT users also felt it was important to upgrade their AT regularly to ensure maximum productivity. One person was very pleased with the outcome when he upgraded his technology: *Knowing that when I did upgrade at times, the improvements I could see were dramatic.* Another was also aware of the importance of upgrading his technology to address postural concerns. He said, *I largely upgraded simply because I knew I could be quicker and also, to a degree, it was concerning my posture problem.*

In fact, one AT user felt that having cutting edge technology was essential for him to compete in the workplace. He said:

I think (that technology) is something that you have to embrace...you do need to update and if you are going to compete with people who have all their physical attributes, then you need cutting edge technology.

At times even upgrading the mainstream technology offered benefits to the person who had previously had to rely on specialized technologies. One AT user stated:

Technology back then wasn't what it is today, like for instance the Access Pack you probably know is now all built-in, so you don't need that cumbersome extra software package.

Those who worked in environments where there was a well-established infrastructure of technology reported that mainstream technology advancements such as e-mails, online schedules, and mobile phones also have contributed to their comfort and efficiency.

Most technologies have a limited lifespan, and it is important to consider what the user is to do when their technology becomes outdated or becomes unreliable. One resourceful AT user, anticipating the imminent collapse of his outdated AT, seized an opportunity to purchase an upgraded version of his AT when the platform technology in the workplace was being upgraded. This extended the life of his AT and ultimately his work efficiency.

RECOMMENDATIONS FOR SERVICE PROVIDERS
Reliability of the Technology

Once the AT user receives his or her technology, many are left to fend for themselves with ongoing technologic difficulties. Although many individuals with disabilities are resourceful and will derive solutions that work satisfactorily for them, others find it more difficult to identify or access suitable resources and if support is not found, over time may start to distrust and then avoid technology.[10]

Rapid developments in mainstream and AT have resulted in compatibility being a persistent problem for AT users.[2] Assistive technologies are mostly developed for small markets by small companies, who frequently lack capital for comprehensive research and development of products. Field testing, where prototypes are tested widely by experienced users, often is not undertaken for AT. This results in problems not being identified until users put them to the test in their own environments.[4] It is, therefore, not surprising that AT users encounter compatibility issues with their technology in the workplace. This issue could be alleviated with better funding or tax incentives for research and development of these products, which would reduce the burden on consumers to perform this function. In addition, large computer software companies need to be more aware of the requirements of specialized technologies so that they can ensure AT users are not excluded from using their products.

Despite the ongoing difficulties AT users experience using their technology in the workplace, there is little mention of this in the AT literature. Inge et al.,[5] in a review of follow-up requirements for three people with spinal cord injury in the workplace, found that twice-monthly follow-up visits identified technologies requiring service and maintenance. However, no studies have been undertaken to date to examine the impact of technical problems on the productivity of AT users. Up until now, AT service providers have largely been concerned with the selection and procurement of technology and have given little attention to the problems AT users encounter in using their equipment. For services to be truly consumer-focused, strategies need to be put in place to ensure that users have the ongoing technical support they require to remain productive members of the workforce. It is evident that AT users who successfully co-opt people to help them deal with technical problems are better able to use their technology in the workplace. However, it is also clear that AT users would benefit greatly from contact with other users, as they often experience similar difficulties with software conflicts and using unreliable technology. Ongoing contact with other users would provide AT users with opportunities to support each other, troubleshoot, and identify useful technical assistance. Some examples of user listservs include the following:

- Voice Users Mailing List: Offers hints and tips and solves many of the most common problems voice users face (*http://voicerecognition.com/voice-users/*)
- Cat-lst: Created for people with vision impairment to discuss computers and assistive technology (*http://groups.yahoo.com/group/cat-lst*)
- Jaws for Windows: Dedicated to the discussion of issues related to using JAWS, a screen reading program (*http://www.wdev.net/oldjfw*)

These listservs provide one way for AT users to be connected with each other so that they do not have to deal with technology performance issues in isolation.

The long-term effectiveness of the AT user is dependent on his or her technology remaining viable. Service providers, employers, and funding bodies require an understanding of the difficulties AT users encounter with aging technology. Furthermore they need to be aware of the potential conflicts between mainstream and specialized technologies when computer systems are upgraded so that issues can be dealt with proactively. A system of follow-up or review can assist AT users to address these challenges[4,6,13] and remain productive in the workplace in the long term.[5] In addition, better processes are required in the workplace to ensure AT users are adequately consulted before mainstream systems are upgraded. Because upgrades are likely to occur every 2 years, it is important that a process is in place to advise the AT user of impending upgrades so that they can work with IT personnel to explore alternative AT options and investigate possible compatibility issues before the change is implemented. Funding also needs to be allocated so that AT users can update their technologies when systems are upgraded.

AT users highlighted the value of having a technology backup in the workplace. People who rely on specialized AT benefit from having alternative options available to ensure ongoing productivity, when their specialized technology is inactive, being repaired, or temporarily crashes. To date, the value of alternative technologies has not been widely acknowledged and discussed in the AT literature; however, they are often identified as being important by consumers. Booth reported that AT users preferred having dual access methods to alleviate fatigue and to replace the primary access method when it becomes inoperable.[3] Further research is required to understand the value of these backup technologies to AT users and their productivity in the workplace. Currently service providers are primarily concerned with identifying technologies in terms of the tasks they are required to perform specified tasks. However, it is clear that further consideration needs to be given to the length of time the user is likely to be working at the task . Alternative technology options allow users to vary their input method and also allow them to maintain productivity when their technology fails. Consideration also needs to be given to the particular dynamics of the workplace milieu, which includes the supportiveness/attitudes of coworkers, supervisor/employer, and IT personnel.

Accessing Technical Support

Technical support is crucial to AT users.[1] However, despite technical support being a significant issue for AT users and their employers, to date only a few procedural models acknowledge the need to set the equipment up in the workplace and provide ongoing technical support.[1,4,7] Apart from identifying a need for a network of technical assistance,[9] little is understood of the nature and amount of support required to enable AT users to be productive in the workplace. Many AT users who had easy access to IT support in the workplace valued this support. For these users IT personnel were involved in the installation and ongoing support of the technology in the workplace; however, the quality of this support varied. Although IT support was readily available when difficulties were being experienced, AT users felt that some difficulties could have been prevented altogether with forward planning and testing before upgrades were implemented. IT support tends to be more readily accessible in larger organizations; however, over half the AT users in this study were either self-employed or employed in small organizations, without access to ongoing IT support. In these situations, support was provided informally by "superusers," IT-literate friends, or alternatively purchased. It is essential that AT users have access to good IT support. To be effective, IT personnel need to be familiar with the specialized technologies being used and how to resolve typical technical difficulties. In addition, they require ready access to specialist information or AT personnel who understand the unique nature of the technology and can assist them in resolving difficulties peculiar to the specific technology being used. If the workplace is not large enough to have its own IT personnel, AT users need to be able to offset the ongoing expenses of technical support against their income so that they can afford to purchase the support they require. AT users also require information about responsive repair and maintenance services[12] that have experienced personnel to assist them as required.

AT users felt also that after-sales support was important to ensuring their technology remained operational. Because day-to-day compatibility issues present one of the greatest challenges to AT users, it is important that those using a number of technologies together purchase all products from one supplier. This removes uncertainty about who is responsible for the technologies' ability to work together effectively. After-sales service is often the first thing to be sacrificed when suppliers are squeezed to provide a competitive quote. As a consequence, the user is left with ineffective technology and inadequate support. It is important that products are purchased from suppliers who are committed to providing after-sales service and have the appropriate expertise to support products. A list of useful questions when choosing a supplier is listed in Appendix E.

In North America, a system of AT supplier accreditation has been established to assist people in identifying suppliers with appropriate expertise. However, a general accreditation does not provide certainty about which area of AT the supplier has expertise. In many countries, there are only a limited number of suppliers of specialized technology, so the consumer has limited choice about where they can purchase their technology. Although many of these companies are dedicated to the service of AT users, limited resources can sometimes result in limited service. It is especially important to also examine the suppliers' expertise and commitment when purchasing mainstream technologies, such as voice recognition technology. Mainstream suppliers often have varied expertise and, more importantly, limited experience with people who rely entirely on these technologies. Information on suppliers, their expertise, and after-sales support would be useful to AT service providers and consumers. AT information services can generally identify relevant suppliers; however, it would be useful if there were AT consumer Web sites where users could post information about supportive suppliers. Appendix F provides a list of questions to assist AT users in examining whether a supplier will provide them with the nature of information and ongoing support they require.

Having a system that provides a replacement while a troublesome device is being repaired would also greatly assist AT users in maintaining their productivity in the workplace. Some AT suppliers provide a replacement when repairing or servicing a device under warranty. Similarly, AT users are able to hire devices from some suppliers when their AT is down for a long period. In some areas, AT users have the protection of legislation such as the "lemon law" created under the Virginia Warranties Act.[14] This bill stipulates that a device must be replaced or refunded if it is out of service or requires the same repair more than three times in the 12 months after delivery. Legislation of this type certainly provides AT users with protection; however, it would be more useful if resources were available to ensure that AT was more reliable in the first place.

Operating as Efficiently and Effectively in the Workplace

Despite having specialized technologies, AT users were not always able to operate in the same way as their able-bodied counterparts in the workplace. With the growing trend toward open office environments, careful consideration needs to be given to the impact of the environment on technology use. Open offices proved to be a barrier for some users, especially those using voice recognition technologies. Noise dissipation in these offices not only affected the reliability of the technology, it also meant that AT users were conscious of disturbing others when using their technology. AT users who had their own offices, where noise could be excluded or contained, were better able to use these technologies.

The interaction between the technology and the workplace environment is a crucial consideration when choosing an appropriate technology. The Human Activity Assistive Technology (HAAT) model provides a very useful framework for examining this interaction and the potential impact on technology choice because of its emphasis on the human, activity, and assistive technology, which interact in context.[4] As noted by the International Classification of Functioning, Disability and Health (ICF),[15] the context can present facilitators or barriers to the successful use of technology. Furthermore, the environment is considered disabling to a person when it presents barries that limit the person's capacity to function. It is clear then that AT users require the workplace to provide adequate ongoing support for their technology if they are to operate as efficiently and effectively as coworkers.

Another model, *Matching Person & Technology* (MPT),[11] also considers the context as well as the person and technology with the definition of the task or activity as preceding these considerations. The MPT Model, as related to the workplace, has been operationalized as an assessment (Workplace Technology Predisposition Assessment) that gathers perspectives of office technologies from the employee and/or employer and their degree of shared understanding. It is designed to assist employees and employers in identifying factors (as shown in Box 6-1) that might serve as barriers to the use of a new technology in the workplace so that appropriate employee training can be planned, modifications made to the technology, and employees' skills enhanced.

AT users in this study often felt locked into one workstation and unable to use communal facilities, vary their work location, or take advantage of the more flexible work practices. Service providers, therefore, need to focus on the accommodations required by the specific individual at his or her current workstation as well as look at opportunities for creating equity within the workplace by advocating for office environments more conducive to the use of these technologies. Discussions should be undertaken within the workplace to examine how or when the existing technologies will be upgraded and how this can support the further integration of the AT user into the workplace, rather than seeing the

---

BOX 6-1
Workplace Technology Device Predisposition Assessment (WT PA)

The employee form and employer form of the **WT PA** consist of two double-sided forms, each requiring about 15 minutes to complete. They were designed to be used together to ensure the following goals:

- Employee input drives the MPT process
- Employers are helped to consider a variety of relevant influences on workplace technology use
- Different perspectives of employee and employer become evident so that they can be addressed

The **WT PA**-Employee Form and the **WT PA**-Employer Form examine the following areas:

- The technology itself
  - Discomfort, stress, fatigue involved
  - Adequacy of the time needed for training and mastery
  - Similarity of currently used technologies
  - Compatibility with other technologies in the workplace
  - Status provided by technology to users
- Complexity or awkwardness of the technology
- The employee being trained to use the technology
  - Previous success with new technologies
  - Feeling of support toward the new technology
  - Feeling of control about adoption of the technology
  - Possession of skills for use of the technology
  - Preferred method of learning the new technology
- The workplace environment
  - Degree of respect and appreciation toward the employee
  - Adequacy of training time for the new technology
  - Knowledge of the benefits of the new technology
  - Availability of different training methods
  - Adequacy of rewards for mastering the technology
  - Existence of a nonthreatening environment for learning

Data from Scherer MJ: *The Matching Person & Technology (MPT) Model Manual and Assessment* [CD-ROM], ed 5. Webster, NY, The Institute for Matching Person & Technology, Inc., 2005.

AT users' needs as being separate to the technology in the work environment. For example, electronic scheduling, intranet, and e-mail can assist AT users in making arrangements, accessing documents, and communicating efficiently with their work colleagues.

A number of AT users also commented on how technology afforded them flexibility in terms of how and where they could work. AT users require technologies that afford them with the same flexibility as their coworkers rather than further restricting them to a specialized workstation. Given the increasing flexibility in the workplace, it is important that AT users have the capacity to move to other workstations and locations as the work requires. Increasingly as workers are being offered the flexibility to work from home, consideration also needs to be given to providing AT users with the capacity to telecommute. This flexibility assists AT users in a number of ways. First, productivity can continue if the employee has medical issues that require them to remain in bed or close to specialist facilities. Second, users can continue to work at home if they have mobility or transport difficulties. Many people with disabilities find getting to work a demanding and complex task, which adds another stress to their day. Third, AT users can benefit from having access to these technologies at home to increase familiarity and proficiency. Finally, these workplace technologies can also provide AT users with access to computer technology and the Internet for household management and personal development.

To be competitive in the workplace, AT users need to update their technology regularly. This requires keeping up with mainstream technological developments. AT users also felt that upgrading their AT periodically enabled them to function at an optimum. Mainstream and AT continue to provide people with disabilities increased access to employment, as well as ease in performing work tasks.[8] These technologies can ensure optimum integration of AT users by providing them with access to *all* the information pathways and facilities in the workplace. However, the productivity of AT users in the workplace can only be assured if their technologies are regularly updated, as new developments become available.

SUMMARY

This chapter has examined the experiences of AT users when using their technology at work. Technology incompatibilities, lack of IT and product support, open office environments, and being locked into one workstation were the main barriers they encountered. They found the backup support of suppliers and IT personnel to be valuable in establishing and maintaining their technology; those who had flexible systems and backup technologies found these beneficial in enabling them to vary their work method and remain productive. Keeping abreast of mainstream and AT developments was perceived by the AT users as essential to enabling them to compete equitably in the workplace. Service providers should ensure that effective support strategies are in place to support the AT user in the long term. Many of the issues raised in this chapter are not well addressed in the extant literature in this field. This research has highlighted a major gap in the body of knowledge on AT in the workplace.

References

1. Alliance for Technology Access: *Computer and Web Resources for People with Disabilities*. Berkeley, Calif, Hunter House, 2005.
2. Beaver KA, Mann WC: Provider skills for delivering computer access services: an assistive technology team approach. *Technol Disabil* 3(2):109-116, 1994.
3. Booth M: *Access and compatibility issues: a survey of consumers*. Paper presented at the Australian conference on technology for people with disabilities, Adelaide, South Australia, October 9-12, 1995.

4. Cook A, Hussey S: *Assistive Technologies: Principles and Practice*, ed 2. St. Louis, Mosby, 2002.

5. Inge KJ, Wehman P, Strobel W, et al: Supported employment and assistive technology for persons with spinal cord injury: three illustrations of successful work supports. *J Vocational Rehabil* 10:141-152, 1998.

6. Kelker K, Holt R: *Family Guide to Assistive Technology*. Cambridge, Mass, Brookline Books, 2000.

7. Nochajski SM, Oddo CR: Technology in the workplace, in Mann WC, Lane JP (eds): *Assistive Technology for People with Disabilities*, ed 2. Bethesda, MD, AOTA, 1995.

8. Pell SB, Gillies RM, Carss M: Relationship between use of technology and employment rates for people with physical disabilities in Australia: publication for education and training programmes, *Disabil Rehabil* 19(8):332-338, 1997.

9. Schall CM: The American Disabilities Act: are we keeping our promise? An analysis of the effect of the ADA on the employment of persons with disabilities. *J Vocational Rehabil* 10:191-203, 1998.

10. Scherer MJ: *Living in a state of stuck: how technology impacts the lives of people with disabilities*, ed 4. Cambridge, Mass, Brookline Books, 2005.

11. Scherer MJ: *The Matching Person & Technology (MPT) model manual and assessment* [CD-ROM], ed 5. Webster, NY, The Institute for Matching Person & Technology, Inc., 2005.

12. Scherer MJ, Vitaliti LT: Functional approach to technological factors and their assessment in rehabilitation, in Dittmar SS, Gresham GE (eds): *Functional Assessment and Outcome Measures for the Health Rehabilitation Professional*. Gaithersburg, MD, Aspen, 1997.

13. Sprigle S, Abdelhamied A: The relationship between ability measures and assistive technology selection, design and use, in Gray DB, Quatrano LA, Lieberman ML (eds): *Designing and Using Assistive Technology: The Human Perspective*. Baltimore, Paul H. Brookes, 1998.

14. Wallace JF, Gilson BB: Disabled and non-disabled: allied together to change the system. *J Prevention Assessment Rehabil* 9:73-80, 1997.

15. World Health Organization: *International Classification of Function, Disability and Health: ICF*. Geneva, WHO, 2001.

Optimizing the Use of Technology in the Workplace

■ "(The AT) has not only reduced my headaches but also improved the quality of the work."—AT Study Participant

When technologies are well chosen and set up, they can have a significant impact on the working life of an assistive technology (AT) user. They can reduce the pain AT users experience from using awkward and demanding postures and movements and contribute to their comfort, satisfaction, and overall productivity in the workplace. This chapter examines the fourth stage of the process of technology acquisition and implementation, namely, optimizing technology in the workplace (Figure 7-1). In the first part of this chapter, the experiences of AT users when using technology to carry out their daily tasks at work will be explored. The second part of the chapter provides service providers with an understanding of the importance of optimizing the use of technology and details strategies that can enable users to take full advantage of their technology. The aims of this chapter are to examine AT users' (1) discomfort and pain when using technology and strategies to address this, (2) understanding of the technology and how this affects use, and (3) experience of learning to use their technology and how their training needs are best met.

■ USER EXPERIENCES

Personal Discomfort and Pain

Experience of Discomfort and Pain

Across disability groups and ages, many AT users experienced personal discomfort and strain when carrying out their work tasks. A number of the participants commented that they became fatigued during the day and experienced muscle discomfort and pain. One participant said:

> *The only thing I'm finding at the moment is when I'm doing a lot of typing, my neck and shoulders tighten up.*

In some cases it was the employer who was most concerned about the employee's posture and approach when working. One employer commented:

> *I was aware that she was keying with just one finger and her positioning seemed rather stressed to me, and I felt she'd be getting a lot of wear and tear on her muscles and, you know, she might get some sort of contractures and problems as she got older, with all the stress she was putting on her body.*

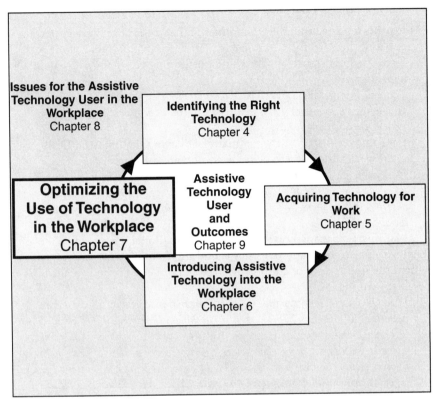

FIGURE 7-1 ■ Stages of choosing and integrating technology into the workplace.

Participants also expressed concern about the long-term implications of effortful and repetitive actions. One participant commented on his current access method:

My neck used to only go when I'd used it (the mouth stick) all day. Now if I only use my neck for 3 hours, it starts to hurt, even an hour or so.

His concern increased after meeting a person who had to have a plate in his neck due to the wear and tear of mouth painting for 27 years.

That sort of taught me a lesson, that if I don't be very careful, I'm going to finish up exactly like him. So all those stories that you think 'will never happen to me,' well it was going to happen and I was getting lots of pain, so I just realized I had to be careful.

Some participants were prepared to endure significant pain over an extended period without investigating the cause or exploring solutions. One participant with cerebral palsy who had been experiencing crippling pain in his neck when using the computer commented on how he had postponed seeing a doctor despite the level of pain he was experiencing:

To be honest, it really frightened me because I never had pain like that before and (next time) I don't think I would put up with it for that long without going to see a doctor.

Addressing Discomfort and Pain

Participants reported that the ergonomics of the workstation were important in customizing their AT for effective use. Participants and employers repeatedly discussed the importance of addressing positioning issues to reduce pain. One participant stated:

> I haven't been getting as much back pain lately. It might be a simple thing (like positioning the monitor) that is more effective (than the technology itself), and the most important thing so far.

For some participants it was a matter of having the time and flexibility to set up the workstation and to position equipment for comfort.

> I was given plenty of choice about my actual physical location, how I wanted to set up my desk, what size or which desks of those that were available I wanted to have, how to configure them. So I was able to set myself up, you know, really quite comfortably fairly quickly.

Many participants reported having an occupational therapist (OT) to assist them with positioning and that they found this helpful. One participant highlighted the importance of addressing the ergonomic issues and recalled his experience with the OT:

> I had OTs as case workers and, really, getting that independent advice was really important in a lot of ways, making sure that things were right. The OT knew about ergonomics and posture, and those are more important, to be honest. You know the technology is a minor thing when you're aware of what's available. And you know it forces you to consider your posture, because you are willing to shortcut....and a bit of professional advice too, there's no better...You know you just don't ask yourself all the questions that need to be asked.

In some cases, the awkward postures adopted by the AT user at his or her workstation prompted the employer to investigate alternative equipment. One employer observed: *He was struggling away with an ordinary computer and he used to work like this* (employer demonstrated a hunched posture to the interviewer). *It was just ridiculous.* Some participants found that the size or arrangement of the technologies often necessitated an alternative desk. One participant had an adjustable desk so that she could adjust as her postural needs changed from day to day. She felt that this adjustability was a very important part of her technology set-up as it ensured that she was comfortable and effective throughout the day. Other participants purchased additional equipment to position devices or to support their bodies. They found that this helped to reduce pain and discomfort and increased their efficiency and endurance. One participant reflected on the value of the wrist support:

> I don't get so tired in the hands any more...Actually I'm starting to use my left hand more now and I haven't really timed myself that much but I think I seem to be doing a lot more typing than I used to.

Some participants highlighted the value of labor-saving strategies, such as macros, which decreased the demands of effortful or awkward input methods. One stated:

That's a pretty important part of what I do, using the macros. In terms of efficiency, in terms of sort of ease of use— I mean the less I use my neck, the more comfortable I'm going to be all day.

A number of the participants commented that they tried to modify their technology to meet their specific needs as inexpensively as possible. Often this was because they were paying for these modifications themselves or relying on the goodwill of volunteers (workmates or friends) to make equipment or work on the software. These modifications were often undertaken in isolation, without information about readily available products. Consequently users often developed inefficient solutions, as illustrated in this quote:

I needed a double control or an Alt key, and just push this mechanical lever, hold the Control down and then move it up. Obviously it's very slow and cumbersome, but at the time I'd never really used a computer much, so I didn't know about (software solutions) or anything like that.

Participants also found it useful to alternate between technologies to reduce the strain of using one method continuously for specific tasks that they find difficult. Other users were forced to explore alternative technologies when it became clear that their current methods were resulting in significant pain or discomfort. One participant recalled the point at which he recognized the need to explore alternatives:

When I nearly wanted to throw the typewriter out the window about 40 times a day, because I was sick and tired of the pain.

Some participants found voice recognition technology an enormous benefit as it required less effort and allowed them to vary their posture. One participant commented: (voice recognition software) *has...significantly lengthened my working life.*

Understanding the Technology

Participants tended to use only the basic features of their technology and were often unaware of how their technology could be further customized to improve their effectiveness. Trial and error and chance learning were common modes of acquiring knowledge about features of the technology. A number of the participants knew of things they wanted to customize but did not know how to go about it. One participant reflected on the difficulty he experienced in trying to find shortcuts in the following statement: *I often find if a program has got shortcut keys, they're not well advertised and nobody knows about them.*

In some cases, because the IT person set up the technology, the user was unaware of the current settings. One participant did not receive the manual for his equipment and was not even aware of its features. Some had tried and failed in attempts to customize their AT, and so had abandoned further attempts. Frequently, when technology was upgraded, users had to recustomize or reestablish shortcuts, and many reported that they had not had time to learn how to do this. For one participant, the only thing stopping her using macros was knowing how, as reflected in her comments:

I guess the other thing I should really try and get on top of is (that) *we changed over from WordPerfect to Word this year. It's just the macro features that I haven't really got the hang of yet. If I learned to use those more, perhaps that would reduce the number of keystrokes.*

Participants who were aware of the features and capabilities of the technology frequently used their knowledge to improve their effectiveness. One participant noted that it was important to fully understand the capabilities of the technology to use it effectively:

The first step is to find out exactly what you can do, and then start looking at ways to improve it. In terms of efficiency, in terms of ease of use, the less I use my neck, the more comfortable I'm going to be all day, particularly now that I'm getting more familiar with technology, knowing what it can and can't do. I can identify what the computer can do for me and find out ways to use it.

The more sophisticated the program, the more difficult it was for the user to understand its features. Two of the participants using voice recognition technology found it frustrating and hard to understand and train, and thus were limited to using only the basic functions:

It's frustrating training at times. I've gone through some of the general training with the manual, just reading the different material they have in there, and done a lot of that, but there's still a lot that has to be trained with commands.

Knowing people who can modify and customize AT was also considered very useful. Participants were resourceful in finding people to make splints, customize voice recognition technology, or modify a keyboard. AT users who had strong links with a rehabilitation setting or supplier appeared to be able to find the expertise they sought. One participant said:

It's very important to have someone who can convert your ideas into fact and that's what I'm saying. As I said before, once you define your need, then you've got to work out who can fill that need and you've got to get them to fill it.

Learning to Use the Technology

Participants learned to use their technology via a range of means. Some had contact with AT service providers who demonstrated basic features while others consulted computer-literate friends. Without this informal support many of the participants would have floundered as illustrated in this quote:

Well I have a couple of very computer-literate friends who I can call on occasionally to give me a hand, other than that it's sink.

Many taught themselves through experimentation, using the manual, or completing online tutorials. Yet a certain level of technologic proficiency and confidence was required for this approach to work effectively. One participant tells of his approach to learning in this quote:

Trial and error...yeah. Finding there was something we wanted to do, try and do it, if it doesn't work, open the book and work it out or make a phone call back to the suppliers and say we want to do this, how do we do it, and they'll often help us out.

Some received training from the supplier, whereas others accessed specialized training services or facilities. Some of the participants were very resourceful or fortunate in accessing training that would have otherwise cost them dearly. One participant told of his fortune in this quote:

> They (suppliers) *put the system* (voice recognition software) *on and they gave me some basic tutoring on it, which was excellent...they threw that in for free with the system because it was such a new, novel idea and it was so interesting for the person themselves who hadn't had work in this area before. But it's about a hundred and fifty dollars an hour for tutoring.*

Those who were introduced to their technology through specialized training found this useful. However, as noted previously, this training was not always tailored to their needs. Participants reported that they preferred learning from someone who could show them how to use their technology in the way in which they were most likely to use it. Those AT users who were able to obtain direct instruction in this way were most successful in finding out what *they* needed to know about the technology:

> We had the initial tutorial and then we made a list of a whole range of things we did and (what) we could use it for...I asked questions pertaining to my particular use requirements and therefore we got answers on that.

Participants also appreciated having easy access to another user who was using similar technology. One participant felt that a fellow user was an important resource, as he could access information at his level and was supported by a user who was familiar with the technology and could overcome problems on a daily basis. Some participants suggested that AT users with extensive experience should be paid to provide support to other users, thus increasing their availability.

> I think that he (the other AT user) is the best resource because he knows a lot of the information that we need....I reckon that having done what we've done, a key role for him is to actually be a consultant for people who want to get back to work with physical disabilities.

Many participants also commented that it would be worthwhile having online access to other users or user groups to share skills and troubleshoot.

Like many of us, the participants preferred to get information and support as they required it. One participant commented on the benefits of informal learning that can occur at work:

> I'll just work with the people to start with and watch them do things and sort of say "how do you do that," look over their shoulder and then do it myself.

In lieu of having other users nearby, participants found the Help screens and online Help in mainstream software useful because it saved them having to plow through manuals, and they appealed for a similar level of support in AT.

Difficulty Meeting Training Needs

Many participants were not able to access appropriate training because of the costs involved. Participants reported that it would cost between $150 and $300 per hour to buy in-home training. They found this cost prohibitive, so they often relied on their own resources to learn about the technology or co-opted help from acquaintances who were interested in the technology. Because of the prohibitive cost of training, some participants relied on their own resources (reading manuals and going through tutorials) to learn how to use the technology. One commented that this was not an efficient way to learn to use the technology:

> *Quite often manuals seem to teach you some of the things that you really don't need to know...and don't show you a whole lot of things that would make life really simple right now.*

Participants who referred to manuals and tutorials for information tended to be computer literate and well placed to take on the challenge; however, they still felt that they would have benefited from further training.

Many participants thought that it was essential to have access to training. One participant emphasized the importance of training, especially for people who have less experience:

> *Training is really important for me but not so important for someone who is a computer buff ... I **need** training.*

One employer commented on the difficulty she experienced in accessing appropriate training for the user. She reported:

> *That was the hardest thing* (accessing appropriate training)...*Looking at who could train these people, and who could support them, and that's why we had to be flexible and a bit creative as to how we went about doing that.*

Some training resources are only available to people who live in certain cities. One user with a vision impairment stated:

> *It would be useful if I lived in* (another city) *so I could access the* (specialist institution)...*because they have the best training scheme and that's free.*

Some participants had access to specialist trainers through product support. Unfortunately, this training was not always tailored to their needs. One participant found the experience overwhelming. He stated:

> *It was good...but I think because he* (the trainer) *was so far advanced on it, he left me well behind because I'm not a reader or a writer. I've only just started learning, so he left me way behind. At the end of it, I thought to myself "do I know how to switch this on?"*

In contrast, another felt that trainers knew the basic features of the technology and how to troubleshoot, but had limited experience using technology on a daily basis. The trainers were, therefore, not familiar with some of the applications that the user required or how to deal with the recurring problems encountered. One participant recounted:

> *I'd moved beyond what he was capable of...they only know how to set it up and to initiate you into the very basics of it all, and to troubleshoot to some extent.*

Relying on Trial and Error and Informal Support Systems

Although most employees can share information and skills about the technology they use at work, the person using AT often has to learn to use their technology in isolation. Participants expressed frustration with the lack of opportunities to share skills or problem-solve with people using similar technology. One participant's quote encapsulates the feeling of many:

> *It's difficult working on your own because you're repeating your own errors... there's not many people that I know who are proficient with (voice recognition*

technology), so I'd really love to have someone just give me a few hours to help me get straightened out on some of these problems.

Many participants who independently learned to use their technology described this as a frustrating experience requiring trial and error. Often they remained unsuccessful, as noted by this comment:

I've been fiddling for ages... trying to use the headset (the headset I use for voice recognition), *to phone directly through the computer...I haven't managed to do that yet.*

This trial-and-error approach was very time consuming, and participants needed to be very resourceful in accessing the information they needed.

Time Required to Develop Proficiency

Considerable variation in the amount of time participants needed to feel comfortable using their AT was reported. Participants who used simple technology frequently felt familiar with it after about 2 days. For some specialized technologies, participants required much longer for learning. Those using voice recognition software reported taking 2 to 4 weeks to learn how to use the software and set up their voice files. One participant with total vision loss reported taking a term (10 weeks) to feel comfortable using all his technology in his new job.

Although a number of participants felt that customizing their technology and developing their skills in using it would improve their efficiency, they did not take time to do it unless they experienced significant difficulties. Participants felt it was difficult to allocate the time required, particularly if they were trying to do it on their own, as highlighted by this comment: *I haven't got time to put into it...so if I need to learn a software package, I need someone to show me how to do it.* Another participant regretted not spending time learning to use the technology in the first instance as reflected in this statement:

And I found that realistically, had I done it (learned to use the voice recognition program) *in the beginning, I would not have purchased the mini-keyboard or the Headmaster and those sorts of things. I would rather have had more time to work with that* (voice recognition program), *preferably with people who had been using it, other paralyzed or partially disabled people who were forced to use that sort of technology and making it work.*

One participant received time in work hours to train herself using the software tutorials, but she experienced difficulties using the training program. Her employer felt that she had abandoned her voice recognition technology because of the time and effort involved in setting up the voice files. She stated: *I think she found that it wasn't worth the effort, so she's back to using the keys.*

A number of participants reported that the difficulty was not having sufficient time at work to customize or learn to use their technology effectively. They felt that their priority at work was to carry out work tasks. Many reported having to use their own time to familiarize themselves with their technology or that their employer *expected* them to learn how to use it outside of work hours. One participant felt that employers were not informed about the time they required to settle into a job using specialized equipment and suggested some negotiation needed to occur to enable the AT user to settle into the position and become proficient with their technology. He said:

> *The bottom line is, they want someone to walk in and be able to sit down and in 3 or 4 days pick up the system,* (but what they need is) *a week or 2 weeks to settle in. What they need is something along the lines of a supportive wage scheme* (to fund this settling in time).

Another participant reported that he set aside time out of work hours to go into work and customize his speed dial system:

> *At work, you don't have time to set up too many things. It's very hard...I occasionally go into work at other times, after hours if I want to practice a bit at something.*

Opportunity to Explore and Practice

Participants felt that they needed more opportunities to explore their technology and practice to feel confident, as reflected in this statement:

> *It's really just practice; the more you use it, the more different things you do with it, the better off you are.*

Many participants reported that having the same technology at home assisted them in customizing and learning to use it:

> *Fortunately, I was coming up for some leave and I took the computer home, the whole box and dice and got it up to a reasonable proficiency at home over my leave. I think that was very, very useful. I think I would have found it very difficult to fit it in, while I was at work, combining work with it.*

A number of the employers were also aware of the benefits of having the employee exploring and developing confidence with their technology at home. One stated:

> *He has this program at home, so this has meant that outside of work hours, he was able to put in all of the extra time he needed to get proficient with the program. He certainly put in a lot of hours.*

Impact of Training Experience on Technology Use

The AT users varied widely in their training experience and use of technology. Some users were self-taught or accessed informal contacts who instructed them on how to operate the essential functions of their technology (dedicated instruction). These users often continued to need support to use their technology effectively or were only able to use their technology to carry out specific work tasks. They were often unaware of other useful features of the technology. Some users who had used technology over an extended period and developed skills with previous devices were able to transfer skills and knowledge to new technologies. Others who received structured training in the use of their technology were able to extend their understanding of the technology by exploring various features and functions they were introduced to in the training. These experienced and well-trained users were frequently able to extend the capabilities of their existing technologies and felt able to actively embrace new technologies as they came onto the market.

▩ RECOMMENDATIONS FOR SERVICE PROVIDERS

Optimization refers to the process of improving the use of technology by adjusting or customizing it to meet the specific requirements of the individual, the tasks being undertaken, the changing environment, and learning to use the technology to carry out the required work tasks. Fine tuning can increase the comfort of the user and improve the efficiency and effectiveness of the technology. Devices can be repositioned, adapted, or redesigned to meet specific requirements. Alternatively, many technologies have features that can be adjusted or customized to suit the individual. Energy-saving options, such as macros or keyboard shortcuts, can also optimize a user's performance. However, optimizing the use of technology requires more than customization of the devices and layout. AT users also need to be familiar with the features of their technology and how to operate them effectively to compete equitably in the work environment.

Why Is Optimization Necessary?

AT needs to be customized to meet the individual's specific requirements and preferences to optimize its use.[34] To date, attention has focused on matching the person and technology before purchase to prevent nonuse,[33] customizing commercial devices that do not meet individual requirements,[10] or both. However, little attention has been paid to customizing technology after purchase to optimize use. Introducing a new technology often presents a number of new challenges to the user. It may require the user to assume new positions or use different actions.[9] Inappropriate selection or incorrect installation of devices can often result in awkward postures and effortful actions.[9] If AT users encounter difficulties in the early stages, they may persist with old habits if devices are not fine tuned to meet their preferences and requirements.[17] Recently, research has raised concerns about the amount of pain and discomfort technology users experience and the long-term implications of this pain.[11,30] Predicting the long-term impact of a new technology during an assessment is difficult. Consequently, many authors advocate for follow-up intervention so accommodations can be adjusted and refined to ensure comfort and promote effective performance.[5,10,21,24,29,35-38] At the very least, technology accommodations should be adjusted to ensure that use of the technology does not result in discomfort and strain with ongoing use.[36] On the other hand, with careful adjustment and appropriate instruction and training, AT users can achieve optimal use of their technology[44] and secure a future in employment.

At the time of assessment predicting some of the demands on the AT user is possible; however, the AT provider should expect to encounter changes and demands in the workplace that require further adjustment and customization. Technology abandonment (or nonuse) can result when changes in the user's performance, activities, or device performance occur, or when environmental obstacles to the technology are encountered and the technology is not able to deal with the changes or obstacles effectively.[36] The user must be as well equipped as possible to adjust his or her technology by being familiar with its features and proficient in its operation.[7,13] Lack of training also has been identified as contributing to the abandonment of technology.[32] Although training has long been recognized as necessary,[7,34] little evidence exists that people are receiving the instruction they require to understand their technology fully. Training should both provide an understanding of the basic functions of the technology and equip the individual to fit and adjust his or her technology for continued efficiency in performance as the requirements of the user, the tasks, or the environment change.[6] Future career opportunities depend on AT users being well equipped to use their technology competently and meet expectations in the workplace.[31] The literature has heralded the importance of choosing the right technology, yet we have little understanding of the experiences of AT users in optimizing the use of their technology in the workplace. This chapter will now examine the experiences of AT users in using their technology and the strategies they found effective in customizing and learning to use their technology.

Discomfort and Pain

Some AT users endured fatigue, discomfort, and pain resulting from poor positioning and use of repetitive and effortful actions to complete work tasks. Furthermore, maintaining awkward postures and using repetitive movements 40 hours a week has an impact on both their day-to-day effectiveness and their long-term viability in the workforce. Notably, AT users are at risk of experiencing ongoing discomfort and pain using their technology,[11,30] as it is difficult for them to adjust their position or vary their actions to relieve strain and discomfort. Sustained postures and prolonged exposure to strain put them at greater risk of developing cumulative stress disorders,[4,25] thus affecting their productivity and ongoing participation in the workforce.

If comfort and ease of use are to be considered when selecting and positioning technology, users should be afforded the opportunity to comment on these issues during assessment. AT users have been found to choose comfort over function when considering technology options,[25] which is often at odds with the priorities of service providers, who may be focused on function.[40] Although issues of comfort may not seem critical when briefly trying a device, comfort can often become a significant issue once the technology is being used continuously. Consequently, follow-up is necessary post-purchase to ensure the technology is allowing the user to adequately meet the daily demands of the workplace and is not putting them at risk of any unforeseen harm or injury.[6] This is especially important, given the hesitation of people with disabilities to draw attention to any difficulties in carrying out work tasks. AT users have been found to be fearful of being fired if they report difficulties and request further accommodations.[28]

Addressing Positioning and Ergonomics of the Technology System
Identifying Symptoms and Warning Signs: Examining Posture

Having employers who are attentive to the potential for injury helps AT users to address these needs. Because AT users have specific requirements and risks, their needs are not always readily identified within mainstream employment or occupational health and safety systems. AT users need to be alert to the risks associated with awkward positioning, repetitive strain, and pain so they can take action and continue to function at their best. Muscle tension and strain can rapidly deteriorate to debilitating pain and reduced function if the cause is not identified and preventative measures are not put in place. Users may benefit from talking with other users or health professionals about their positioning and actions and the long-term implications of persisting in demanding postures or movements. Further research to explore the ergonomics of AT use is needed so that the extent of pain and discomfort among AT users is more clearly understood. This information would allow greater emphasis to be placed on achieving sound ergonomic solutions, rather than on less cost-effective options.

Many people are unaware of the postures they assume when engrossed in work tasks. For this reason, it is useful to ask a colleague to comment on your work posture or alert you when your posture appears awkward. Alternatively, having someone take a photo of the AT user at work can enable the users to examine their posture more objectively. Users could also be encouraged to take note of *when* they are uncomfortable or experiencing strain, *where* they experience the discomfort, and *what* they were doing at the time that contributed to it and if it intensifies or happens more quickly in the coming weeks. Recording this information using self-report scales, such as verbal rating scales, visual analogue scales,[39] or behavior rating scales may assist the users to monitor and report on pain and discomfort.[30] Once they have details, they may be better placed to discuss the cause of the discomfort with their employer, occupational health and safety personnel, doctor, or therapist, rather than having to declare they have reduced work capacity as a result of pain.

Principles of Ergonomics

The design of workstations and computer equipment continues to evolve in an effort to improve the efficiency and usability of devices. Consequently, the fields of human factors research and ergonomics have flourished in recent years with the increasing demand to understand and apply the science of engineering psychology. Although human factors research has traditionally focused on how humans interact with devices or environmental design,[20,22] ergonomics has been primarily concerned with the fit between the individual and the activity being performed, and aims to promote health and productivity as well as safety and comfort.[9] Human factors research has contributed much to the increasing usability of technologies; however, whenever devices are designed, they are done so with the broadest application in mind. This results in solutions that, although suited to most people who are likely to use it, inevitably do not fit all end users. Not surprisingly, people with unique requirements experience difficulty using devices. Many people with disabilities do not interact with equipment in a way anticipated by the designers.[22] This means that they rarely find the *ideal* product but rather, after weighing up the advantages and disadvantages of various options, select one that has the best potential to suit their requirements. The adjustability of the solution is therefore critical in ensuring that the user can adjust and fine tune the device to fit them.

As people have moved from physically active, multidimensional jobs to unidimensional office work,[18] ergonomics has contributed greatly to maintaining the well-being and efficiency of the workforce. Extensive occupational health and safety legislation and policies have ensured that workers are provided with equipment suited to their needs and are educated about the ergonomics of workstations, as well as how to prevent injuries. As in ergonomics, AT service providers have long appreciated the importance of good posture. Traditionally they have been more focused on the human factors (i.e., fitting the device to the capabilities and limitations of the user rather than the ergonomics, how well the technology fits with the tasks to be undertaken, etc.). Consequently the technology may not always enable the user to carry out the range of activities they wish to achieve or the outcomes the activities demand. With the focus on fitting the technology to the user, sometimes the process may not encourage the dynamics of technology use to be fully explored. As a result, users are not always aware of the importance of the ergonomics of use or equipped to monitor their posture and actions while using their technology in a variety of activities. AT users must be informed about ergonomic principles so they can apply them to their own technology use and work situation. Many of the general principles of good ergonomics apply equally well to AT users, as outlined in Box 7-1.

The ergonomics of AT users are sometimes compromised because these individuals are often seated in a wheelchair, which results in standard furniture and arrangements being inadequate. In addition, AT users frequently use a limited range of actions, which can limit the variability of working postures and actions available and where things can be positioned. Consequently, three ergonomic elements require particular attention: (1) the user's position, (2) the position of work tasks, and (3) the position of the keyboard, keys, and objects.

The User's Position. To maximize abilities and enable the best possible motor control, AT users need to be seated in a stable position with appropriate support. This applies whether they are using standard or customized seating. Most wheelchair seating is designed with an emphasis on providing a comfortable,

---

BOX 7-1

Ergonomic Principles for Technology Use

- Avoid awkward postures such as bending forward or extending the neck
- Maintain joints in neutral positions, head in the midline, upright back, upper arm relaxed beside trunk
- Avoid prolonged static positions; use supports if required to hold a static position for a long period, vary posture with other activities or take frequent rest breaks
- Avoid awkward or effortful repetitive actions
- Take frequent breaks

relaxed sitting posture. However, when engaged in work tasks, people sit more upright, moving their center of gravity forward toward the activity.[10] This is achieved by rotating the pelvis forward and keeping the spine straight, a position often facilitated by office chairs that have a static or adjustable forward tilt in the seat. However, people in wheelchairs, without tilt in space, compensate for the lack of adjustability in their seating by flexing the spine, often being required to hold this awkward and unsupported posture for protracted periods. This posturing places them at risk of injuries, such as strained ligaments, back pain, and disc herniation.[18] An active work posture also requires controlled use of the arms and head. This places further demands on the spine and, in some cases, the user requires additional trunk support to perform these movements comfortably and accurately. The user's seating must be examined in terms of its adequacy to support work activities and additional adjustments, features, or supports provided to ensure the user is comfortable and well supported in an active sitting posture.

   The Position of Work Tasks. Because wheelchairs are higher than standard chairs, further modifications need to be made to enable the AT user to function in the workplace:

- The height of the desk: When using hands to access a keyboard, a tray, desk, or laptray, it should be at a height that allows the keyboard to be placed at or slightly below elbow height. This ensures that minimum shoulder abduction is required to access the keyboard, thus allowing a more controlled and efficient approach to the keyboard. When using head access, the keyboard should be elevated so that the user is not flexing or extending the neck unduly to access the keyboard.
- The angle of the work surface: As discussed previously, without an adjustable seat angle, additional flexion is required of the upper spine to work on a flat work surface. An angled work surface (10 to 20 degrees positive angle) reduces the need for neck flexion and makes it easier to read and write. However, a sloped work surface also can make it difficult to place objects. Therefore it is important to identify the tasks to be undertaken and observe the resulting positioning issues before deciding if this is appropriate.
- Position of the monitor: The monitor should be positioned so that the user can view the screen while holding his or her head in a neutral position. According to the United States Department of Labor, Occupational Safety and Health Administration (www.osha.gov/SLTC/etools/ computerworkstations/ index.html), the monitor should be directly in front of the user with the top of the screen no higher than eye level and approximately 20 to 40 inches (50 to 100 cm) from the eyes, and tilted 10 to 20 degrees (where the top of the screen is further back than the bottom of the screen). A swivel monitor or a monitor on an arm allows it to be repositioned for specific tasks.
- Placement of the keyboard: The keyboard should be placed an appropriate distance from the user to keep the shoulder in a neutral position when the user's hand is held over the center of the keyboard. Similarly, when the person is using a head pointer or mouthstick, the end of the pointer should be over

the keyboard when the client holds it in a neutral position. The client should not be required to use trunk flexion to reach the keyboard.

- The keyboard should be centered within the user's active range of movement. If the person is using one hand, the keyboard should be centered around that shoulder so that he or she can access the entire keyboard with ease, without having to cross the midline or use lateral trunk flexion to reach areas of the keyboard.
- The keyboard should be angled in the vertical plane to best meet the requirements of the user. Some people, especially those using mouthsticks or head pointers, find that they can see the keys and access the upper rows more easily if the keyboard has a positive tilt (i.e., the back of the keyboard is higher than the front of the keyboard) of between 10 to 20 degrees. A stronger angle may be required if the user has limited shoulder flexion, control over movements, or is using a head pointer. People with limited wrist extension or wrist pain often use a negative vertical tilt (i.e., the front of the keyboard is higher than the back of the keyboard), which allows them to maintain the wrist in a neutral position.
- When using one hand, access is often improved if the keyboard is angled in the horizontal plane to allow more efficient access to the left and right extremes of the keyboard. This follows the natural arc of movement of the arm when the shoulder is internally and externally rotated, (i.e., when using the right hand, the bottom left hand corner of the keyboard is closer to the body [Figure 7-2]). This position reduces the amount of shoulder abduction and flexion, thus enabling more distal control. For those with different movement patterns, the angle should reflect the arc of movement the user has available to them. Some users find they have better access with the keyboard angled in the opposite direction.

These factors can significantly affect the (1) user's tone and posture, (2) efficiency of approach, (3) ease of access to all keys, (4) accuracy and speed of access, and (5) level of fatigue the user experiences.

Position of Keyboard, Keys, and Objects. The layout of the keyboard and objects on the desk should make the best use of the user's movement capacity:

- Range of movement: the area they can reach comfortably
- Control of movement: the area they can reach reliably
- Accuracy and speed: the ease with which they move between locations

The range of movement of the user and the control they have within that range will determine the optimum workspace. The ability to make discrete movements within that area will determine what type of activities can be undertaken in that area.

The area of user control will vary in different areas of the workspace. A one-handed person (right-handed) is likely to benefit from a workspace arranged according to Figure 7-3.

Important or frequently used objects or keys should be located in the primary access areas.[16] Unfortunately the QWERTY layout, standard on computer keyboards, does not take into consideration that fingers vary in strength, dexterity,

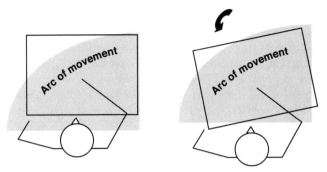

FIGURE 7-2 ■ Keyboard positioned to optimize use for one-handed user.

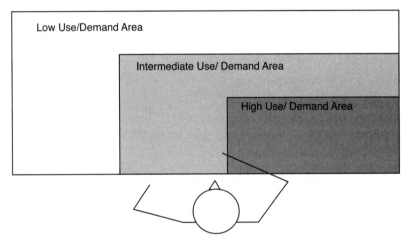

FIGURE 7-3 ■ Workspace allocation for a one-handed person.

and susceptibility to fatigue.[43] In 1943 Dvorak keyboards were designed to provide an alternative ergonomic layout (i.e., placing frequently used keys in accessible areas of the keyboard) for 10-fingered typists[43]; however, despite this layout being shown to be easier to learn and achieve greater speed and accuracy, QWERTY remains the industry standard. Alternative layouts are also available for one-handed typists and single input methods such as typing stick, mouthstick, and head pointer. These keyboards have been found to be useful in decreasing errors and increasing speed,[3] as well as assisting users who keyboard for long periods or need to increase their productivity. For users who are reluctant to change from the familiar layout, important keys or those in an awkward position can be relocated to be more accessible (e.g., backspace).

Thus the user's performance must be examined closely to determine the optimum height of the desk, layout of the workstation, position of the monitor and keyboard, and location of frequently used objects or keys.

Accessing Expertise

A number of the AT users' more ergonomic positions alleviated pain and discomfort. Although some AT users experiment with various configurations until they are comfortable, others find it useful to have a service provider assist them to set up their workstations. The goal of ergonomics is to establish the best fit between the person and the activity to promote health, safety, comfort, and productivity.[9] Professionals who have traditionally provided ergonomic assessments in the workplace are occupational therapists, physical therapists, and related health and safety professionals. It is important for AT users to identify if they have access to ergonomic advice within the workplace or to access AT service providers with the appropriate expertise to help them achieve an ergonomically sound set-up. The ergonomics of the workstation may require periodic review to ensure that it remains appropriate for the individual, the tasks being undertaken, and the environment as abilities, responsibilities, and demands in the workplace change.

Augmenting the Existing Technology Systems

Optimizing technology can sometimes require that additional equipment be acquired to allow the technology to be positioned more effectively, to allow the position of the technology be adjusted in response to daily requirements, and to provide the user with additional support or alternatives to relieve discomfort and maintain productivity throughout the day. Frequently, the size or arrangement of new technologies necessitates a larger or alternative desk. An adjustable desk that allows its height to be altered enables AT users to position the desk to suit the nature of tasks undertaken. For example, reading and writing require a higher desk than keyboarding. Additional positioning equipment, such as a monitor arm, can be useful for effective positioning, such as adjusting the position to provide more comfort, or pushing it away to allow more desktop space. Some AT users may find that once they are established with their technology, they have a need for additional support, such as forearm or wrist supports, to enable them to keyboard for longer periods or to provide additional support in the latter part of the day. Some users find it useful to have two different technologies between which to alternate, to reduce the strain of using one method continuously, or use technologies best suited to specific tasks that they find difficult. At some point, if a technology has been adjusted or customized extensively and is still found not to be suitable, more appropriate alternatives need to be explored. Accurately predicting the usability of a solution long-term is not always possible, and AT users should be encouraged to seek solutions that fit their ongoing requirements and the demands of the workplace.

Making the Most of the Technology's Existing Features

Understanding technology's existing features and capabilities in order to customize for individual requirements is essential. Without this knowledge, AT users struggle to complete tasks that could otherwise be completed effortlessly. AT users who are aware of the features and capabilities of their technology frequently use this knowledge to improve their effectiveness. For example, time can be saved by using keyboard shortcuts or macros, whereas using features such as "autocorrect" can conserve energy.

Ability to Customize Technology

Unfortunately, an AT user's ability to customize and use his technology effectively can be significantly hampered by lack of information and knowledge, limited access to support, isolation, inadequate time, the complexity and unintuitive design of the technology, and frequent upgrades of the platform computer systems that necessitate relearning and further adjustments. In addition, when IT personnel or other people take responsibility for the technology, the user remains ill equipped to make adjustments as required. AT users with a sound understanding of the features and capabilities of the technology were better able to make the required adjustments. Alternatively, having knowledge of and access to people with appropriate expertise also enables AT users to optimize their use of technology. Although the AT literature has consistently promoted the importance of the AT user understanding his or her technology[7,34] and follow-up and training support,[33,41] little evidence exists that demonstrates people have access to the information and resources they require to utilize their technology fully. Building a "circle of support" is very important, not just for identifying the best technology[1] but also to provide AT users with resources to meet their ongoing needs.[41] AT users found it useful to have access to people who could assist them to position their technology ergonomically, locate a suitable wrist support, build a splint, fix a head pointer, show them how to use shortcuts, and advise them on upgrades and improvements to their technology. Access to these resources varied depending on the system they used to identify their technology initially and where the person worked. However, the reality remains that people using technology in the workplace have ongoing requirements and are best able to adjust and customize their technology when they have access to a wide range and variety of resources. Appendix G details questions AT users can ask themselves when using their technology to determine if they need to further customize their AT system.

Training
Difficulty Meeting Training Needs

Many AT users continue to have individual training needs that remain unmet despite having had their technology for some time. When a user's training needs are not anticipated in the funding package or acknowledged by the employer, the user is left to rely on his or her own resources, using trial and error, or consulting friends to understand the technology. Many teach themselves through experimentation, wading through manuals, or completing online tutorials. Novice users who are self-taught or only understand basic aspects of their technology do not extend their technology beyond essential functions and are likely to require ongoing support. AT users who are computer literate or well informed about resources are best equipped to build on their existing skills when approaching new technology and resolve training issues independently. Less-confident AT users with limited technology experience or expertise find experimentation frustrating and time consuming. AT users are often isolated from other users and, therefore, have limited learning opportunities where they can benefit from the experience of others. In the absence of this incidental learning, AT users are forced to seek the informal support of friends and colleagues. Without this support many AT users flounder. However, even with this support, many, especially those with little experience or expertise, remain uninformed about key aspects of their technology. Users continue to comment that they are not able to ask "the right people the right questions."[17] Skill development that relies on "miscellaneous sources cannot be said to provide a secure foundation for planning, development, or long-term viability" (p. 30).[19]

Training is an important part of the process, but we do not as yet have a clear understanding of what constitutes adequate training.[45] Models have been proposed that outline the range of knowledge required to use AT. To date, not enough is known about what is required to ensure that the user is competent and confident in AT use and how this outcome can be measured.

Need for Tailored Training

All users, especially novices, benefit from structured instruction. However, even those who are technically proficient appreciate the benefits of training. Training permits users to understand the features of their technology and use these to accomplish work tasks. Even users with little prior experience are able to become functional users with structured training. Although training has been consistently identified as a critical need in the literature,[8] AT users continue to find it difficult to access appropriate training. Current systems for accessing training on specialized products, such as learning support from a supplier, clearly fall short of meeting the diversity of need. Mainstream training facilities also have not been found to accommodate the needs of people with disabilities.[26] Training is said to be more effective if it is targeted at the specific learning needs of the user.[15,35] Without an appreciation of the diversity of AT users' experience and skills, appropriate training systems cannot be developed. AT users vary in their level of experience and often require highly individualized training according to their abilities, experience, and work-related goals.[23] Furthermore, not all users have a desire to be technical specialists. Although some users have an active interest in technology and require an in-depth understanding of the application of the technology, others are novices and require a gentle introduction. Furthermore, whereas some prefer to be totally self-reliant in their use of technology, others prefer to supplement their defined knowledge using external advisors or people in their support network.[2] Valuable training time must be used well and designed to meet the immediate needs of the user. An understanding of the current skills and experience of the user, the tasks to be performed, and the existing demands and supports in the work environment will assist the trainer to identify the level of knowledge required by the user and the key functions that they need to understand. The objectives of the training should be developed in conjunction with the user and stated explicitly[2] to ensure that the sessions are targeted appropriately and that the user is active in the learning process.

An essential component of any training program is finding the right balance between providing success and challenges to the learner. Learners need to feel they are achieving knowledge and skills and have their accomplishments acknowledged. A well-structured learning program can identify manageable objectives and maintain an "optimal challenge balance."[2] Initially, new users should not be overwhelmed. However, as users gain experience and develop proficiency, their learning needs will continually become more sophisticated. This necessitates that a "spiral curriculum" be developed[35] to ensure that the ongoing learning needs of the user will be addressed. Training programs need to be developed to meet the needs of novice, intermediate, and advanced users,[10] so that users can select the most appropriate program and have access to higher level training as their skills develop.

Traditionally, users are provided with information on the technology's capabilities and how to perform various functions. Users are assumed to be able to integrate this theoretical and procedural knowledge and apply it to their own situations. However, AT users also need to learn specific functions related to their work application (practical knowledge), how to fix problems, learn about other functions as the need arises (know how), and be able to contextualize their learning (a knowledge of being) to use their technology effectively.[2] Thus, training should not only introduce the specific features of the technology related to the person's immediate needs but also should ensure that the user understands the *logic* of the technology and is comfortable with exploring its capabilities. The challenge is to design a program that allows the user to acquire an appropriate mix of knowledge. It is important that, in addition to instruction or demonstration, users be afforded a range of learning experiences, such as experience-led discussion, drill and practice, experimentation, modeling, skill sharing, and real-time problem solving and troubleshooting to ensure that they are able to build on their existing knowledge and integrate learning into their work practices.[2] Providing users with access to a range of learning experiences also can ensure that the user's ongoing learning needs are met. AT service providers could also benefit from examining the literature on systems of training support found to be effective when introducing mainstream technologies into the work environment. Strategies suggested by Martinko, Henry, and Zmud,[27] such as associating the technology with prior successful experiences, pretraining that provides explicit levels of usage success, implementation plans that eliminate early failures and ensure early successes, and opportunities for modeling successful users are all likely to assist AT users in making the most of their technology.

If users do not feel comfortable with the technology or are not able to develop an understanding of how it operates, they may need to access additional training at a later stage after they have mastered the basic functions and are ready to understand the technology more fully. Service providers also need to acknowledge the AT user's previous experience and level of comfort with technology when making recommendations. Those with past experience may well be able to transfer skills onto the new technology and thus require less training support. The more interest AT users have in technology, the more likely they are to extend their technology possibilities. Where possible, arousing the user's interest in technology and empowering them to continue their understanding and skill development are vital to their success. This exploration allows them to adjust their technology to meet their current needs, extend their technology to meet their ongoing needs, and be self-sufficient in the workplace. Appendix H has a series of questions to guide AT users in learning to use their technology.

User Support

In addition to training, AT users value having access to other users who have an in-depth understanding of the technology, its features, and its application. Previous studies have confirmed that people's computer skills improve while at work, suggesting that on-the-job training assists in developing mainstream computer skills.[31] Many of us have developed computer skills by watching others and picking up skills from our work colleagues. Having access to others who use the technology on a daily basis and have acquired a detailed understanding of it provides users with an efficient way to learn more about their technology. On-line access to other users or user groups has already been promoted for information sharing during selection[15]; however, its role in skill sharing and troubleshooting remains underutilized but would be invaluable in addressing users' sense of isolation and providing ongoing learning support.

The AT user's innate interest in technology also appears to have an impact on willingness to explore the technology possibilities in terms of extending their current technology as well as exploring potential technologies. Service providers can often put these AT users in touch with other individuals or groups of AT users. Where possible, service providers can also promote mechanisms for AT users to keep in contact with each other through directories, listservs, user groups, and discussion lists. Service providers should be wary not to generalize the experiences of these people onto all AT users. Although some users only require access to user groups for skill sharing, other users may require more formal training support.

Time Requirements

Many users find it difficult to allocate the time required, especially in the initial stages, to become familiar with their technology. As found in previous studies,[23] the less experience an AT user has with technology, the more time he or she is likely to require to become comfortable. In addition, some technologies have steep learning curves, requiring the user to invest many hours to master the technology before they can be proficient with it at work.[15] Some employers are aware time is required to become familiar with new technology; however, many expect the user to become proficient in his or her own time. Educating the employer about the time required to become proficient with the technology and predicted proficiency rate was identified by Turner et al.[42] as essential to promoting good long-term job satisfaction and employer-employee relations.

Technology at Home

Having the same technology at home facilitates the exploration and use of all facets of the technology, and has been found previously to support its effective use in the workplace.[12,23] Users, particularly those who are not familiar with technology, have been found to prefer to practice in private while gaining skills and confidence without being observed.[22] In this study, the AT users relied on the goodwill of the employer or resourcefulness of the service provider to allow them to take the AT home, despite this being a necessity. In 1991, a policy letter was introduced to special education in the United States that clarified the right of children with special needs to take their technology home from school.[14] Similar legislation is necessary for workers to ensure that they can take advantage of this strategy to optimize their work performance.

SUMMARY

This chapter has identified the structures that are important for effective AT use and strategies that ensure AT users are able to master and optimize their use of technology in the workplace. Factors that limit AT use, such as discomfort and pain, limited knowledge of the technology's features, and the complexity of the technology, have been highlighted. The amount of time required for training, limited work time available for mastery, cost of training, and limitations of the training provided resulted in an overreliance on trial and error and informal support networks and a sense of isolation. AT users enhanced their use of technology by addressing the ergonomics of the workstation and customizing the technology to address individual needs and strategies. Other key strategies included tailored training and learning support, as well as opportunities to practice using the technology and to explore its features away from work demands. Currently, the success of AT users can most easily be attributed to their experience and resourcefulness rather than to a well-structured system of training support.

References

1. Alliance for Technology Access: *Computer and Web Resources for People with Disabilities.* Berkeley, Calif, Hunter House, 2005.
2. Andrich R, Besio S: *Critical Factors Involved in End-Users' Education in Relation to Assistive Technology.* Milano, Italy, European Commission, Deliverable 6 of the EUSTAT study, 1999.
3. Anson D, George S, Galup R, et al: Efficiency of the Chubon versus the QWERTY keyboard. *Assistive Technol* 13:40-45, 2001.
4. Anson D, Lawler G, Kissinger A, et al: Efficacy of three head-pointing devices for a mouse emulation task. *Assistive Technol* 14:140-150, 2002.
5. Bain BK, Leger D: *Assistive Technology: An Interdisciplinary Approach.* New York, Churchill Livingstone, 1997.
6. Bazinet G: Assistive technology, in Karan OC, Greenspan S (eds): *Community Rehabilitation Services for People with Disabilities.* Boston, Butterworth-Heinemann, 1995.
7. Beaver KA, Mann WC: Provider skills for delivering computer access services: an assistive technology team approach. *Technol Disabil* 3(2):109-116, 1994.
8. Behrman MM: Assistive technology training, in Flippo KF, Inge KJ, Barcus JM (eds): *Assistive Technology: A Resource for School, Work and Community.* Baltimore, Paul H. Brookes, 1995.
9. Burwell CM: Ergonomics, in Bain BK, Leger D (eds): *Assistive Technology: An Interdisciplinary Approach.* New York, Churchill Livingstone, 1997.

10. Cook A, Hussey S: *Assistive Technologies: Principles and Practice*, ed 2. St. Louis, Mosby, 2002.

11. Cowan D, Turner-Smith A: The user's perspective on the provision of electronic assistive technology: Equipped for life? *Br J Occup Ther* 62(1):2-6, 1999.

12. Decker CA: Technical education transfer: perceptions of employee computer technology self-efficacy. *Computers Human Behav* 15:161-172, 1999.

13. Dowler DL, Hirsh AE, Kittle RD, et al: Outcomes of reasonable accommodations in the workplace. *Technol Disabil* 5:345-354, 1996.

14. Galvin JC: Assistive technology: federal policy and practice since 1982. *Technol Disabil* 6:3-15, 1997.

15. Galvin JC, Donnell CM: Educating the consumer and caretaker on assistive technology, in Scherer MJ (ed): *Assistive Technology: Matching Device and Consumer for Successful Rehabilitation*. Washington DC, American Psychological Association, 2002.

16. Goosens G, Crain S: *Augmentative Communication Assessment Resource*. Birmingham, Alabama, University of Alabama, 1986.

17. Gradel K: Customer service: what is its place in assistive technology and employment services? *Vocational Rehabil* April:41-54, 1991.

18. Hermenau DC: Seating, in Jacobs K (ed): *Ergonomics for Therapists*. Boston, Butterworth-Heinemann, 1999.

19. Hunt HA, Berkowitz M: The background and setting, in Hunt HA, Berkowitz M (eds): *New Technologies and the Employment of Disabled Persons*. Geneva, International Labour Office, 1992.

20. Jones ML: Human factors and environmental access, in Olson DA, DeRuyter F (eds): *Clinician's Guide to Assistive Technology*. St. Louis, Mosby, 2001.

21. Kelker K, Holt R: *Family Guide to Assistive Technology*. Cambridge, Mass, Brookline Books, 2000.

22. King TW: *Assistive Technology: Essential Human Factors*. Needham Heights, Mass, Allyn & Bacon, 1999.

23. Lash M, Licenziato V: Career transitions for people with severe physical disabilities: integrating technology and psychosocial skills and accommodations. *Work* 5:85-98, 1995.

24. Lazzaro JJ: *Adaptive Technologies for Learning and Work Environments*, ed 2. Chicago, American Library Association, 2001.

25. Leger D, Halpern M (eds): *Cumulative Trauma Disorders*. New York, Churchill Livingston Inc., 1997.

26. Lupton D, Seymour W: Technology, selfhood and physical disability. *Soc Sci Med* 50:1851-1862, 2000.

27. Martinko MJ, Henry JW, Zmud RW: Attributional explanation of individual resistance to the introduction of information technologies in the workplace. *Behavior Information Technol* 15:313-330, 1996.

28. McNeal DR, Somerville NJ, Wilson DJ: Work problems and accommodations reported by persons who are postpolio or have a spinal cord injury. *Assistive Technol* 11:137-157, 1999.

29. Nochajski SM, Oddo CR: Technology in the workplace, in Mann WC, Lane JP (eds): *Assistive Technology for People with Disabilities*, ed 2. Bethesda, MD, AOTA, 1995.

30. Patterson DR, Jensen M, Engel-Knowles J: Pain and its influence on assistive technology use, in Scherer MJ (ed): *Assistive Technology: Matching Device and Consumer for Successful Rehabilitation*. Washington DC, American Psychological Association, 2002.

31. Pell SB, Gillies RM, Carss M: Relationship between use of technology and employment rates for people with physical disabilities in Australia: publication for education and training programmes. *Disabil Rehabil* 19(8):332-338, 1997.

32. Phillips B, Zhao H: Predictors of assistive technology abandonment. *Assistive Technol* 5:36-45, 1993.

33. Scherer MJ: *Living in a State of Stuck: How Assistive Technology Impacts the Lives of People with Disabilities*, ed 4. Cambridge, Mass, Brookline Books, 2005.

34. Scherer MJ: The impact of assistive technology on the lives of people with disabilities, in Gray DB, Quatrano LA, Lieberman ML (eds): *Designing and Using Assistive Technology: The Human Perspective*. Baltimore, Paul H. Brookes, 1998.

35. Scherer MJ, Galvin JC: An outcomes perspective to quality pathways to the most appropriate technology, in Galvin JC, Scherer M (eds): *Evaluating, Selecting, and Using Appropriate Assistive Technology*. Gaithersburg, Md, Aspen, 1999.

36. Scherer MJ, Vitaliti LT: Functional approach to technological factors and their assessment in rehabilitation, in Dittmar SS, Gresham GE (eds): *Functional Assessment and Outcome Measures for the Health Rehabilitation Professional*. Gaithersburg, Md, Aspen, 1997.

37. Sowers JA: Adaptive environments in the workplace, in Flippo KF, Inge KJ, Barcus JM (eds): *Assistive Technology: A Resource for School, Work and Community*. Baltimore, Paul H. Brookes, 1995.

38. Sprigle S, Abdelhamied A: The relationship between ability measures and assistive technology selection, design and use, in Gray DB, Quatrano LA, Lieberman ML (eds): *Designing and Using Assistive Technology: The Human Perspective*. Baltimore, Paul H. Brookes, 1998.

39. Straker L, Jones KJ, Miller J: A comparison of postures assumed when using laptop computers and desktop computers. *Appl Ergon* 28(4):263-268, 1997.

40. Tate DG, Riley B, Forchheimer M: Enhancing the appropriate use of assistive technology among consumers and caretakers, in Scherer M (ed): *Assistive Technology: Matching Device and Consumer for Successful Rehabilitation*. Washington DC, American Psychological Association, 2002.

41. Treviranus J, Petty L: Computer access, in Olson DA, DeRuyter F (ed): *Clinician's Guide to Assistive Technology*. St. Louis, Mosby, 2001.

42. Turner E, Barrett C, Cutshall A, et al: The user's perspective of assistive technology, in Flippo KF, Inge KJ, Barcus JM (eds): *Assistive Technology: A Resource for School, Work and Community*. Baltimore, Paul H. Brookes, 1995.

43. Weiss T, Chan C: Computers and assistive technology, in Jacobs K (ed): *Ergonomics for Therapists*. Boston, Butterworth-Heinemann, 1999.

44. Wessels RD, Dijcks B, Soede M, et al: Non-use of provided assistive technology devices: a literature overview. *Technol Disabil* 15:231-238, 2003.

45. Wielandt PM, McKenna K, Tooth LR, et al: Post discharge use of bathing equipment prescribed by occupational therapists: what lessons to be learned? *Phys Occup Ther Geriatrics* 19(3):49-65, 2001.

CHAPTER 8

Issues for the Assistive Technology User in the Workplace

■ "I was getting to the stage where my first 3 months had been extended for another 3 months and I was still having difficulties. There were problems with accuracy and, basically, once I started to become acquainted with different forms of equipment and things like that my accuracy improved and my work improved to the extent that I was able to be appointed."—AT Study Participant

As highlighted in the above quote, without the "right" technology, assistive technology (AT) users experience difficulty in sustaining employment. Many people with disabilities struggle on, using ineffective methods for fear of drawing attention to their difficulties or making additional demands on the workplace. Although *gaining* employment is often the focus of discussion in the literature, it is *maintaining* employment that is difficult for people with disabilities.[9] It is, therefore, important to develop a greater understanding of people who have been successful in gaining and maintaining employment[9] and what has contributed to their ongoing success. This chapter examines the fifth stage of the process of technology acquisition and implementation, namely dealing with ongoing issues in the workplace (Figure 8-1). The first part of this chapter explores the experiences of AT users in making requests for technology in the workplace and their willingness to advocate for themselves. In addition, their expectations of employers and their experience in using supports to facilitate negotiations in the workplace are presented. The nature of the workplace, and employers and coworkers' awareness of issues and expectations of AT users are then discussed. Finally, the implications of these for professionals providing AT services will be examined.

■ USER EXPERIENCES

Some participants felt comfortable discussing their technology needs with their employer(s), whereas others were not only uncertain about their needs, but also felt uncomfortable with placing demands for additional resources on their employer.

Advocating for Themselves

Despite employers having an expectation that the employee would initiate requests, many AT users expressed reluctance to advocate for themselves for fear of seeming to be demanding or otherwise compromising their employment

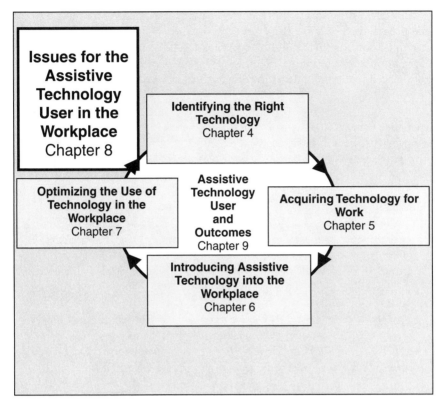

FIGURE 8-1 ▪ Stages of choosing and integrating technology into the workplace.

opportunities. The following quote summarizes the feeling of many: *When you're just starting your job, you don't want to make too many waves.* Having to initiate requests placed the participants in a difficult position, given that they reported feeling disinclined to inconvenience anyone or make demands of the employer. When reflecting on having to initiate requests, one participant stated:

> *You see that's why I feel very vulnerable because...I'm always terrified of telling my boss of what needs I have...because I have to compare with a person who is capable ...You see what I'm getting at?*

Some employers also acknowledged the difficulty employees with a disability experience in advocating for themselves. One employer stated:

> *People are often reluctant to access reasonable adjustment. Some people prefer to think that they don't really need that. I guess it's part of our history of being as able as one can with a disability and fighting away, and then it's like saying yes, but I do need some special things. Some people have personal difficulty with acknowledging some of that.*

Participants were routinely expected to take responsibility for finding out about the AT available and how they could access it, even when they were unsure of their needs or the processes involved. Regardless of their degree of autonomy or willingness to advocate for themselves, many participants found it difficult to approach their employer and advocate for their technology needs when they were not aware of the technology options available to them. Thus, a lack of information about available technologies coupled with a reluctance to request them placed many individuals in the position of having inadequate support in the workplace.

Participants were more inclined to advocate for themselves if they had prior experience using AT in the workplace, were confident in identifying their technology needs, were in positions where they had autonomy, or had previous positive experiences with advocating for themselves. These participants reported that they were happy to advocate for their technology needs, but they needed to be independent and persistent to achieve the results they required. One commented:

> I think that people are busy, they've got priorities, they can't always think of me when they've got lots of things to do. So it's probably up to me. If I speak up, I've generally had results in the past.

Other participants held positions of responsibility and felt that they would be expected to have the skills required to identify their needs and appropriate equipment. One said:

> I am a middle manager and the Department would expect nothing else from a middle manager. The Department will provide support for people who don't have the same sort of savvy and who demonstrate that they need more support. But I haven't needed it and I'm not a shrinking violet so if I want something, I'll seek it out.

Use of a Service Provider to Facilitate Negotiations with Employer

A number of the participants appreciated the assistance they received from service providers (from either a human resources [HR] department within the workplace or an external employment service) to assist them in negotiating within the workplace and liaising with the network of resources. Apart from being familiar with the funding systems, legislation, and how to negotiate with employers, these service providers were able to justify the accommodations in a language that the employers understood. One participant explained:

> Well, when I first started, Management and Workplace Health and Safety Department (there was an OT there), they were open, they were making the approaches. It wasn't a matter of them keeping their distance and waiting for me to ask for something. They were looking at ways. So even if nothing else, the fact that the people were open and actually coming to me instead of me hounding them...put out the welcome mat (and) made me feel more comfortable and looking more at solutions to problems, rather than just the problems themselves.

Many participants welcomed the intervention of an outsider, as they were often hesitant to initiate a request to explore other options. One participant explained:

> I guess I'm just the kind of person who works with what I've got unless there is a significant problem or someone suggests something different that is worthwhile exploring.

Other AT users found the assistance of a service provider helpful, as it reduced the stress on them and limited the things they had to be responsible for. One participant commented:

It put a lot less strain and stress on me until I knew someone else was actually organizing everything.

Employers also acknowledged the value of having an independent person to identify the needs of the AT user to ensure the information was unbiased. One employer stated:

It would be also better if you have it (information on the technology required) *from an independent person because it's always very easy for anyone to initiate information for their benefit...It would be far better if you have outside information from an independent resource.*

Expectations of Employers

Participants felt that employers needed to be better informed about *how* to meet the needs of their employees. They felt that accessing networks of information and resources would assist the employer in this process and relieve the employee of some of the burden of having to provide all the information on resources and technologies to the employer. One participant commented:

It would be a lot easier if the employer has all that information. Knowing who to contact or other bodies like...to ensure the process is available or how to undertake that process.

Employers also acknowledged a need for knowledge of technologic possibilities. One stated:

People don't recognize the possibilities if they're not aware of the assistive aids that people might access, then they're not going to be able to explore those with the particular employee, so you need to have some sort of knowledge of all the possibilities.

Another employer felt that access to information about technology options would also allow the employer to take responsibility for initiating action. He said:

It is harder for the employee to receive all the information and dump it on the employer; it would have been a lot better if the employers get the information from outside sources to pass on to the employee...it's important from the top down rather than the bottom up because you are going to confront the barriers as you go up. Its much harder going up than it is going down.

One participant suggested the need for a network that employers could access to assist an employee with an acquired disability who was not familiar with the system or resources available. He stated: *I would really hope there'd be mechanisms that employers would avail themselves of for advice and networking and support for people* (requiring AT).

Nature of the Work Environment

The AT users worked in a range of work environments that differed with respect to awareness of the AT users' requirements and the supports available to assist them in identifying and addressing their technology needs. Participants who were self-employed were responsible for identifying and purchasing their own AT, whereas those working in small organizations found they were mostly receptive to requests for technology accommodations. Local or state government departments used various resources to meet the AT users' immediate needs, whereas national government agencies had well-defined processes for addressing the AT users' immediate and ongoing requirements.

Coworkers and Employers' Awareness of Issues

Apart from those who were self-employed or doing contract work, all the participants were in open employment and worked with people who had limited experience of working with people with disabilities. Most of the participants stated that people at work were friendly and supportive; however, the work environments varied in terms of their responsiveness to individual needs. Employers and coworkers had a low level of awareness of the AT user's requirements. More importantly, many were not even comfortable discussing these. Some employers felt uncertain about what to expect of a person with a disability and how best to approach them. This is summarized well by the following quote from an employer:

> It is interesting because when he first came I had no idea what to expect. I wasn't trained. I wasn't given any information on his needs…it would have been better if the employee had told the employer what their needs are…I wouldn't know if I was infringing on his privacy (by asking him).

Participants commented on a need to acknowledge the lack of exposure of employers and coworkers to these issues and to accept their limited understanding. One participant commented:

> I need to be mindful of where they are at…this is quite a large step that they have made as a private enterprise in having a person with a disability working in a medical environment. For that initiative we have to accept that as it is…I need to be patient with that to some extent; yes it is very, very frustrating but I guess it will just take time to dawn on them that I can't do anything until my environment is how I need it to be.

Employer Approach

The employers all expressed an eagerness to be fair and accepting of the person with a disability and to respond to their requests for accommodations (budgets permitting). Although some employers had some initial hesitation in providing money for equipment, antidiscrimination policies in the workplace facilitated their acceptance of the employee's disability and the subsequent accommodations made. One participant recalled:

> I suppose this is possibly one of the best places to work for as far as their policies are concerned. I know there's a lot of people with amputations who have lost their jobs.…I'm lucky that I not only have a job but they have bent over backwards to provide whatever is recommended for me.

Employers generally saw themselves as having responsibilities to the employees with disabilities. One employer summarized these responsibilities and commitment in the following statement:

> As a manager, you have a responsibility to make sure your staff are in circumstances, regardless of whether or not they have a disability, that are going to optimize their capacity to work well, and disabilities run into that continuum. So you've got a responsibility to make sure their particular needs are able to be accommodated within their workstation area, or their office, or whatever it might be.

In many workplaces, however, there was a lack of clarity about the process of review required to identify the necessary accommodations. One technology user had been employed for 10 months and raised issues within the research interview that his employer was not aware of:

Employer: *Basically I leave it to him to discuss what it is he needs, so I am taking the lead from him...*

Employee: *I probably have to write a proposal.*

Employer: *Well that's right. A proposal is discussed and if I more or less agree, then I go straight to the person above me. That's how the process works here. But to be honest we haven't initiated any proposal, have we? There's something wrong there.*

When offered an opportunity to reflect on what had happened to date, this employer became aware that the employee had not yet initiated any requests.

Workplace Processes

Workplaces dealt with the needs of the AT user in one of three ways. A number of workplaces responded to issues when and if the AT user raised them. These work environments could be called *responsive* work environments. Others were more active in encouraging the employee to make requests and supporting them in the process. These could be referred to as *supportive* work environments. The third type of work environment was proactive in anticipating the needs of the AT user by providing regular reviews and discussing changes in the work environment and their potential impact on the AT user. These are *proactive* work environments. Each of these environments and the implications for the AT user will now be discussed.

In responsive work environments, AT users were generally expected to identify and articulate their needs to the employer. They were also expected to know what technology existed, what they needed, where to purchase the device, how to use it, and how to integrate it into the workplace. Because employers were generally uncertain of the best way to deal with AT issues, they often placed the onus on the employee to advocate for himself or herself in the workplace. This placed unrealistic expectations on the AT user. Employers expected them to have knowledge of AT and to be able to identify and utilize generic and specialist resources. Many participants reported that the employer relied on them to determine their needs and initiate requests. Employers also confirmed that they depended on the employee to identify suitable technology and to provide information to the employer on what was required. One employer said:

Basically I leave it to him to discuss what it is he needs, so I am taking the lead from him...but he hasn't indicated to me that he has needed that sort of assistance at this point in time.

This particular employee had indicated that he had unmet needs in the interview with the investigator of this study; however, he had not informed his employer of these needs.

Many employers in these workplaces also had an expectation that the person with the disability knew all about specialized equipment and perceived the employee to be an expert in the area, even if the employee did not have extensive knowledge about AT. One employer's statement represented the attitude of many employers: *He* (the employee) *is the expert on access issues, but also, you know, equity issues and things like that.* The employee referred to in this statement did not perceive himself in this way. Having a disability did not automatically make him either an access or AT expert.

Supportive workplaces recognized that the employee had a need, sought appropriate resources, and brought in expertise to assist with meeting the employee's technology needs. One employer commented on the resources used to assist with identifying the employee's need:

R: *What difficulties, if any, have you encountered in this process?*

Employer: *Nothing. The person from Human Resources Department and* (the service provider) *from the employment agency are the people who did it.*

R: *So you brought in specialists.*

Employer: *Yes. There isn't anyone within this section who is really capable.*

In these workplaces, the employer worked with the employee and sought additional expertise to identify technology needs and potential devices, and to assist with implementing the technology solution. These environments responded to issues as they arose and were keen to support the AT user in the process.

Other participants commented that their workplaces were very proactive in ensuring that they had exactly what they needed to work effectively. One participant recalled his surprise when the workplace anticipated his needs before the computers were upgraded. He commented: *I was going to approach them about it, but they approached me first.* Again when this person changed jobs, the new workplace also was proactive in accommodating his technology needs. These workplaces often had an equal employment officer (EEO), who assisted the AT user in identifying issues that were likely to impact on their work performance. EEO or HR officers also tried to anticipate the impact of workplace changes on the AT user and were available to the user to periodically review their setups. One officer explained her role in the following quote:

Usually we would be looking at what's the price of the equipment, what are the suppliers, gaining approval for funding, placing the order, ensuring the equipment is installed, and that the staff member's properly trained, knows how to operate it, and if he just needed support. What we have been doing subsequently though is following up...Is the equipment needing maintenance? If so, getting that organized.... We advise them when they're issued with their equipment, that if they have problems to contact us and, if they leave the department, to let us know and it's returned to us...We have a quarterly review where we would check on major pieces of equipment that are still being used and that they still meet the staff members' needs.

The AT users felt comfortable discussing their work performance and technology needs with these officers, as they were not in the AT user's immediate line of command. One participant explained the value of these officers in the following quote:

We have an equal opportunities office and probably federal (government) *is ahead of most state organizations in that respect of providing people with equipment and helping people to obtain information about what is available. And I think that it's been an excellent initiative.*

▓ RECOMMENDATIONS FOR SERVICE PROVIDERS

Advocating for Themselves

Generally, employers assumed that AT users would initiate requests for accommodations and take responsibility for identifying their needs and finding out about the AT available, regardless of their degree of autonomy, knowledge of resources, or willingness to advocate for themselves. Research suggests that "leaving it up to the worker" to identify their needs is common practice, especially in small businesses.[6,16] However, many users did not initiate requests because they were concerned about drawing attention to themselves, uncertain how their situation could be improved, or anxious that their request would have a negative impact on their employment. AT users with prior experience in making requests or who held positions with managerial responsibilities felt better able to initiate requests and access appropriate resources. Even with this knowledge and experience, however, these AT users felt that they had to be independent and persistent to achieve good outcomes.

For many people with disabilities, maintaining employment is dependent on their ability to advocate for themselves.[10] Concerns have been raised that people with disabilities are forced to deal with obstacles in the workplace alone. This is made especially difficult if they are reluctant to advocate for themselves and employers are uncertain of the employee's needs and how to address them. Some feel that education of the employee provides the key to empowering AT users in the workplace.[3,15] Although it might be reasonable to expect that education will assist employees with a disability to address their needs, it has not been found to resolve the issue. Rumrill and Garnette provided people with disabilities with education and social skills training to assist them in discussing reasonable accommodations with employers. They found that those who received the training knew their rights and were better able to implement accommodations in the workplace than their untrained counterparts.[10] For AT users who prefer to be responsible for their own destiny and who have the personal resources to take on the workplace system, developing skills in self-advocacy would be advantageous. However, AT users who are reluctant or unable to assert themselves may require the support of mentors or service providers to assist in identifying needs and negotiating with employers. It is important to recognize that employees with disabilities are expected to self-advocate, to be and remain knowledgeable about AT options, and to stay current in what they need to know to do well in their job. These demands may be an excess burden on people who already experience challenges in their worker role.

Use of a Service Provider to Facilitate Negotiations with Employer

Some AT users found the support of a service provider invaluable in assisting them to anticipate their needs, access resources, and negotiate with the employer. This assistance was useful in stimulating action and reducing the stress experienced by the employee who was trying to address needs. Employers also valued having a service provider involved, as they felt that a specialist could provide an independent review of the employee's requirements and navigate unfamiliar resources to achieve a good outcome. It is important to be aware of the difficulty AT users experience in either acknowledging their needs, identifying appropriate AT, or advocating for their rights. Despite the emphasis on consumer involvement, very little exists in the literature that examines the views and opinions of AT users regarding the issues they face in selecting and using technology in the workplace. AT users in this study varied in their level of interest, familiarity with and knowledge of technology, and preferred level of involvement in the process of exploring options. Service providers, therefore, need to recognize the experience, knowledge, and expectations that users bring to the process and provide services that reflect this diversity.

A broad system of information and services is required to provide AT users with their preferred level of information and assistance. For experienced or knowledgeable AT users, direct access to information systems is necessary to allow them to initiate requests and drive the process. Alternatively, inexperienced users or those with limited interest in or knowledge of technology, value the personalized assistance of a service provider. This assistance enables them to identify potential options and resources and source appropriate funding. Service providers also have a valuable role to play in informing and supporting employers and HR personnel so that they are equipped to recognize their responsibilities and source information on options and resources. It is incumbent upon service providers to be sensitive to the preferences of each AT consumer and informed about the resources and processes within workplaces so that they can adequately assist users to acquire the technology they require and facilitate the development of processes within the workplace to monitor its ongoing effectiveness.[2,7]

Expectations of Employers

At present, there is a dearth of literature addressing the issues of employer and employee expectations. The current study has identified the need for further research into employer perceptions, expectations of the employee, and the AT user's willingness and ability to fulfill these expectations. Scherer and Vitaliti also have called for research into expectations of employers and the availability of support.[12] There appears to be uncertainty as to who is responsible for initiating and driving the process. Although employers think that AT users will bring issues to their attention, it has been noted that there is a reluctance on the part of the AT user to raise issues. It is often difficult, however, for employers to raise issues if they feel ill equipped to deal with them.

Both participants and employers felt that employers needed a better understanding of technologic possibilities and resources. One way in which employers are supported is through the Job Accommodation Network (JAN), which was established in North America to provide employers from a range of industries with information on accommodation options.[5] Inquiries to this network have largely been related to the needs of people who are seeking to maintain or improve current employment, with only 10% of inquiries related to new appointments.[5] It should be noted that with the majority of calls to this network being in relation to musculoskeletal injuries to the upper limb,[5] the service is largely being used to address the needs of existing employees who develop an injury or disability rather than those with a disability who are attempting to enter the workforce. However, as proposed by the AT users in this study, access to appropriate information networks would assist employers in undertaking a review process and working with employees to address their specific needs.

Some propose that a united approach, focused on educating both the employer and employee about their rights and responsibilities, is also required to facilitate the integration of the AT user into the workplace.[10] However, knowledge alone does not ensure that employees' accommodation needs are met.[18] Employers also need to facilitate open communication between themselves and the workers, demonstrate a commitment to supporting and maintaining AT users in the workplace, and develop clearly articulated policies and processes for addressing the ongoing needs of AT users.[18] By initiating discussion, employers can reduce the burden on AT users to advocate for themselves. The need for open communication was a consistent issue discussed by people with disabilities, coworkers, supervisors, employers, and HR and union personnel in a series of focus groups conducted by Westmorland et al.[16] Communication within the workplace was highly valued by the focus group participants who also recommended better communication between services.

Although an accepting work environment goes some way to enabling AT users to feel welcome in the workplace, employers also need to show a commitment to supporting and maintaining AT users in the workplace. Research suggests that while placement rates of people with disabilities in employment may be encouraging, continuity of employment or advancement is difficult to achieve.[14] Commitment to AT users in the workplace is best evidenced in establishing explicit processes, which enable employees to discuss their ongoing needs with their employer, access appropriate resources, and identify suitable accommodations.[10] Review processes need to be in place to ensure that the technology accommodations continue to meet the employee's needs and determine if any further customization or training is required. This process could easily be tied to current workplace review mechanisms, such as an annual appraisal. It is also important that workplace accommodations are seen as occurring beyond the point of entry into the workforce and strategies are developed to address changes in the individual's skills and abilities, work responsibilities, and workplace technologies and practices. AT users also need to be empowered to address their ongoing needs by being informed about impending changes in the workplace and having clear processes for action.

It has been noted previously in research undertaken in small workplaces[6] that many do not have suitable policies and processes to support people with disabilities.[16] Many of the principles and processes concerning occupational health and safety or workplace disability management are equally, if not more, applicable in addressing the needs of people with long-standing impairments and AT users who are entering the workforce.[18] Limited research has been undertaken to investigate employees' perceptions of organizational policies and practices.[18] One study examined the impact of organizational behaviors on work disability prevention and management. Its findings showed four organizational policies and practices as being important to workers following carpal tunnel surgery. These included people-oriented culture, safety climate, disability management, and ergonomic practices.[1] Clearly, organizational policies and practices of this nature, especially disability management, would greatly assist in addressing the issues AT users experience in the workplace. Disability management is defined as "a pro-active, employer-based approach to: a) prevent and limit disability; b) provide early intervention for health and disability risk factors; and c) foster coordinated disability management administrative and rehabilitative strategies to promote cost effective restoration and return to work" (p. 88).[18] Although disability management practices primarily aim to manage safe and early return to work, it is equally suited to managing the ongoing needs of AT users.[18]

Nature of the Work Environment

It is clear from the comments of the AT users in this study that they generally felt accepted by their employers and coworkers, but that these sentiments were not always translated into appropriate action. Because of their limited experience with people using AT, employers and coworkers were unclear about the needs of the AT user and were uncomfortable about approaching them to clarify these. As noted previously, this process can be facilitated by developing appropriate policies and processes that enable the ongoing needs of AT users to be addressed within the workplace.[18]

Although antidiscrimination policies exist and employers felt a responsibility to be fair, lack of established processes often placed the onus on the AT users to define their needs, identify and access appropriate resources, and advocate for themselves in the workplace. The value of legislation for ensuring people with a disability are accepted into the workplace has been highlighted repeatedly in the literature.[4,8,11,15] However, the findings of this study concur with concerns raised by Schall[11] that employers and employees were hesitant to discuss the true needs of the individual where responsibilities and processes are unclear. Structures need to be put in place and processes made explicit, if the needs of AT users are to be adequately addressed.

Three types of work environments were identified in this study: responsive, supportive, and proactive environments. Each of these environments dealt with the AT user's needs in different ways (Table 8-1). It is important that service providers are aware of the nature of the work environment and work with the AT user to ensure their ongoing success. AT users who are prepared to actively self-advocate are likely to achieve good outcomes, regardless of their work environment. Similarly, a proactive work environment is likely to support good outcomes for AT users, even if they are reluctant to initiate a request.

TABLE 8-1

Characteristics of Different Workplace Environments

TYPE OF WORKPLACE	CHARACTERISTICS OF WORKPLACE ENVIRONMENT
Responsive	Require employee to identify/articulate own needs
	Expect employee to initiate request to employer
	Assume employee knows what technology is available
	Rely on employee to access appropriate resources
	Have limited understanding of what is required to install, use, and maintain technology
Supportive	Acknowledge employee's AT needs
	Encourage employee to report needs when they arise
	Seek appropriate resources to address needs
	Engage service providers with appropriate expertise
	Work collaboratively with employee to identify AT and implement solution
	Ensure technology is adequately installed
Proactive	Have workplace consultant (EEO or HR officer) who provides support and is outside of employee's line of command
	Have workplace consultants take responsibility for investigating suitable technology options
	Anticipate needs in advance of appointment, job change, or computer upgrades
	Have established regular review mechanisms

The acceptance of people with disabilities in the workplace is optimized if the people in the workplace are aware of and sensitive to the needs of their coworkers.[17] However, as evidenced by the comments of AT users in this study, although an accepting environment resulted in employers being responsive to requests, it did not ensure that employees raised their concerns. Some contend that the responsibility rests with service providers or AT professionals to ensure that the needs of AT users are identified and addressed.[13] Others, however, prefer that mechanisms within the workplace are developed or extended to incorporate the needs of AT users.[14,16] Employers need to be aware of the difficulties AT users experience in both identifying their needs and advocating for themselves. They also require an understanding of the needs of AT users and information on suitable accommodations and resources. Systems for periodic review of AT users' needs should also be established and AT users informed about these processes. Service providers can support AT users in responsive environments by empowering them to advocate for themselves. AT users need to understand their rights, as well as appreciate how to activate processes within the workplace and use strategies and resources to achieve a good outcome.[10] Service providers may also need to provide ongoing support to both the employers and employees to ensure these processes work well and that they have adequate information and resources to address AT users' needs. Similar support also may be required for AT users who are self-employed or engaged in contract work.

Supportive workplaces allow employees to define their needs and identify suitable accommodations. They tend, though, to respond to issues as they arise and do not necessarily have structures in place for periodic review or to anticipate the impact of upcoming changes in the work environment. These workplaces go some way to addressing the AT user's needs; however, there is no guarantee that issues are identified or addressed in a timely manner. Service providers can assist in these environments by providing employers with a deeper understanding of AT users' ongoing needs, how to recognize problems when they arise, and how to establish reliable systems for periodic review. Some AT users also may require ongoing support to make use of review systems and be persistent in making requests. Service providers also need to promote the development of proactive work environments by educating employers on the needs of AT users, assisting the employer to establish effective processes, and providing input into policy development.

Proactive work environments have officers who are responsible for periodically reviewing employee needs and anticipating the impact of impending workplace changes. A particular advantage of this system is that these officers were viewed by AT users as colleagues, which allows AT users to discuss openly their ongoing needs. In addition, the use of existing business or natural workplace supports improves the inclusion of people with disabilities in the workplace and reduces the alienation they may experience when using specialized supports.[14] Employers also have been found to have a very positive view of the use of existing workplace systems to support employees with disabilities.[14] Specialist AT service providers may have a role in this system by providing information and support to these officers.

SUMMARY

This chapter has outlined the issues encountered by participants in dealing with their AT needs in the workplace. It explored the nature of workplaces, the employers' and coworkers' awareness of the issues, and their expectations of AT users. Additionally, the AT users' willingness to initiate requests for AT in the workplace was examined. The interaction between the AT users' willingness to advocate for themselves and the level of support provided by the workplace, along with the implications of these interactions for professionals providing AT services, was also discussed. Questions to guide users in promoting the long-term use of assistive technology in the workplace are provided in Appendix I.

References

1. Amick B, Habeck RV, Hunt HA, et al: Measuring the impact of organizational behaviors on work disability prevention and management. *J Occup Rehabil* 10(1):21-38, 2000.
2. Bazinet G: Assistive technology, in Karan OC, Greenspan S (eds): *Community Rehabilitation Services for People with Disabilities.* Boston, 1995, Butterworth-Heinemann.
3. Behrman MM: Assistive technology training, in Flippo KF, Inge KJ, Barcus JM (eds): *Assistive Technology: A Resource for School, Work and Community.* Baltimore, Paul H. Brookes, 1995.

4. Butterworth J, Kiernan WE: Access to employment for all individuals: legislative, systems and service delivery issues, in Lehr DH, Brown F (eds): *People with Disabilities Who Challenge the System.* Baltimore, Paul H. Brookes, 1996.

5. Dowler DL, Hirsh AE, Kittle RD, et al: Outcomes of reasonable accommodations in the workplace. *Technol Disabil* 5:345-354, 1996.

6. Eakin JM: Leaving it up to the workers: sociological perspectives on the management of health and safety in small workplaces. *Int J Health Services* 22:689-704, 1992.

7. Hirsh A, Duckworth K, Hendricks D, et al: Accommodating workers with traumatic brain injury: issues related to TBI and ADA. *J Vocational Rehabil* 7:217-226, 1996.

8. Lunt N, Thorton P: *Employment Policies for Disabled People.* Moorfoot, England, Research Management Branch, Employment Dept., 1993.

9. Rumrill PD: Employment and multiple sclerosis: policy, programming, and research recommendations. *J Preven Assess Rehabil* 6:205-209, 1996.

10. Rumrill PD, Garnette MR: Career adjustment via reasonable accommodations: the effects of an employee-empowerment intervention for people with disabilities. *J Prevent Assess Rehabil* 9:57-64, 1997.

11. Schall CM: The American Disabilities Act: are we keeping our promise? An analysis of the effect of the ADA on the employment of persons with disabilities. *J Vocational Rehabil* 10:191-203, 1998.

12. Scherer MJ, Vitaliti LT: Functional approach to technological factors and their assessment in rehabilitation. In Dittmar SS, Gresham GE (eds): *Functional Assessment and Outcome Measures for the Health Rehabilitation Professional.* Gaithersburg, Md, Aspen, 1997.

13. Steinfeld E, Angelo J: Adaptive work placement: a "horizontal" model. *Technol Disabil* 1(4):1-10, 1992.

14. Trach PD, Koch LC, Harris J: Employers' and service providers' perspectives regarding natural supports in the workplace. *Rehabil Counseling Bull* 41(4):293-312, 1998.

15. Turner E, Wehman P, Wallace JF, et al: Overcoming obstacles to community re-entry for persons with spinal cord injury: assistive technology, ADA and self advocacy. *J Prevent Assess Rehabil* 9:171-186, 1997.

16. Westmorland MG, Williams RM, Strong S, et al: Perspective on work re-entry for persons with disabilities: implications for clinicians. *Work* 18:29-40, 2002.

17. Westmorland MG, Zeytinoglu I, Pringle P, et al: The elements of a positive workplace environment: implications for persons with disabilities. *J Prevent Assess Rehabil* 10:109-117, 1998.

18. Williams RM, Westmorland MG: Perspective on workplace disability management: a review of the literature. *Work* 19:87-93, 2002.

CHAPTER 9

Evaluating the Effectiveness of Technology in the Workplace

■ "Not everything that counts can be counted, and not everything that can be counted counts."—Albert Einstein (attributed)

As detailed in previous chapters, there are many complexities in selecting and using assistive technology (AT) in the workplace. Consequently, it is difficult to define the success of a technology intervention and determine what contributed to it. The future development of technology interventions and quality services depends on the development of evaluation processes which clearly define expected outcomes and monitor factors which contribute to the success of interventions. Too frequently the evaluation process is directed by the tools available, both standardized measures and generic assessments and most frequently surveys, rather than a clear understanding of the indicators of a quality intervention. Things that are easy to evaluate do not always provide an accurate picture of the overall effectiveness of an AT system. Furthermore, there are important aspects of the system and the process that are difficult to capture and quantify.

This chapter will outline the importance of evaluation in ensuring AT users are well equipped to be productive members of the workforce and discuss the challenges faced in evaluating the effectiveness of technology in the workplace. It will examine the range of stakeholders with a vested interest in AT outcomes and the value of using a consumer-centered approach to evaluating outcomes. The implications of the timing of outcome evaluations also will be discussed. Based on the experiences of the AT users described in previous chapters, this chapter will outline the nature of outcomes required to support the effective use of technology in the workplace. Domains of AT outcome evaluation and current measures will then be described. Finally, parameters for examining existing outcome measures will be provided to assist service providers to select appropriate tools for AT outcome evaluation.

▓ IMPORTANCE OF EVALUATION

To date, many policy makers and funders have been so impressed by the "sexy, glamorous and razzle-dazzle nature" (p. 101)[22] of technology that they have not considered it necessary to evaluate the effectiveness of these devices.[22,33] Similarly, consumers, service providers, and manufacturers also have assumed that technology will automatically improve quality of life.[33] The perceived benefits of technology is one reason that the evaluation of the effectiveness of technology solutions has been slow to take hold.[33,79] Traditionally, the AT industry has largely relied on personal testimonials and anecdotal experiences to validate the impact of technology and services.[21,89] More recently, a plethora of home-grown survey tools has been developed by researchers and services to evaluate specific aspects of AT interventions.[54] Although the benefits of AT are beginning to be documented in the literature,[79] their effectiveness for consumers is not being routinely evaluated.[89]

As devices become more expensive and demand for funding increases, there will be a need to justify expenditure and demonstrate the effectiveness and efficiency of services and devices.[20,40] Consumers also are demanding more information on the relative benefits of devices to assist them in decision-making.[21] In addition, the increasing number and diversity of devices necessitates a more rigorous approach to evaluating their comparative merits.[34,40,79]

Service providers have an obligation to ensure good outcomes for consumers[33] and to maintain and improve the quality of services.[20,33] Knowledge acquired from these evaluations can facilitate market decision-making and the further development of technologies. In addition, evaluations provide evidence of the effectiveness of specific interventions or practice approaches.[33] By continually managing and evaluating services, costs can be minimized and desired outcomes maximized.[21] Evaluation also helps to determine which interventions are effective, for whom, and in which contexts[33,34,54,89] and which may result in additional harm or unexpected outcomes. It also is not uncommon that follow-up evaluations uncover additional or unmet needs.

▪ TECHNOLOGY NONUSE

To date, evidence of the effectiveness of technology interventions has been inadequate.[89] Concern has been increasing in the literature about the discontinued use, or nonuse, of technology.[4,42,58,59,68] Follow-up studies consistently show that 30% to 50% of recommended assistive devices, such as hearing aids, mobility and self-care equipment, are discarded.[84] The overarching factor associated with device discard is a *change in the priorities or needs of the user*.[37,58,84] Factors found to influence continued use of a device are: the performance of the device, consumer involvement in device selection, motivation to use the device or do the task, continued availability of the device, access to meaningful training, information about repair and maintenance, need for a change or to surmont environmental obstacles, and whether the device was seen by the user as effective, reliable, durable, comfortable, and easy to use.[15,69,76,84,92] Psychosocial factors, such as the social acceptability of the device and the degree to which the device benefits the user's performance of and participation in desired activities, have also been proposed as key factors in the acceptance of assistive technologies.[7,42] In addition, the "hassle index," that is, the relationship between the functional gain and the degree of hassle involved in using the device, has been proposed as underlying people's decision to accept or to reject a device.[94]

Technology nonuse has serious repercussions, which include the waste of scarce resources and, more importantly, people with disabilities performing less than optimally. Research on nonuse has addressed assistive devices in general, with mobility and grooming aids being the most nonused or discarded devices.[15,69] Little is known about nonuse of AT in the workplace. Even less is understood about the AT user's level of satisfaction with technology and how these devices affect their performance of activities, participation, and quality of life. Concerns have been raised that service providers lay the responsibility for device discard on the user and do not examine other factors, such as the role of the technology or service provider in nonuse.[16] Many have called for a better understanding of the process of choosing and using technology,[71,84] as well as a closer examination of services involved in the process[31] and how these contribute to technology utilization. Questions remain unanswered more than a decade after they were raised: "Are people getting the devices they need? If they get them, are they using them? What happens when the technology breaks down, wears out, or no longer meets the need? Are the devices making the difference we hoped they would?" (p. 966).[71]

CHALLENGES TO EVALUATING OUTCOMES

Evaluating the outcomes of AT interventions presents many challenges. For example, AT is often provided as part of a number of interventions, and it is therefore difficult to ascertain the degree to which the AT is responsible for the outcome.[20,22,33,38,92] The expanding range of technologies available makes it difficult to define the expected outcomes.[35,40,92] Service delivery is diverse and fragmented, which prevents quality of outcomes and services from being measured in any meaningful way.[20,74] Poor outcomes can result from poor technology or failure at any stage of the process.[33] The difficulty in separating AT from the service context and other interventions results in uncertainty about the outcomes of the devices.[33,79,89] There is also very little standardization across services in terms of the nature of assessments used and information collected.[89]

It is often proposed that the variability amongst AT users and their individual goals makes it difficult for specific outcomes to be evaluated.[20,38,72] When selecting devices, people often have to make compromises, which invariably means that the outcome will not meet their original expectations. People often have to settle on a less-than-optimal device because of the high cost of their preferred device.[72] In addition, an AT user may have a constant level of pain, which makes it difficult for them to evaluate the comfort of a device.[72] A number of variables, such as a past negative experience or an unsupportive application environment, may also contribute to the failure of a technology intervention.[38,82]

THE PURPOSE OF EVALUATING AT OUTCOMES

Traditionally, outcome measurement has been the province of rehabilitation providers and researchers,[33] but it has become increasingly important in decision-making and quality assurance in service delivery.[29] Researchers and rehabilitation providers measure outcomes to establish the efficacy of interventions,[53] to provide reports for litigation purposes, to inform management and funding bodies about services, to refer to other providers, and to benchmark against other services.[29,89] Numerous standardized tools have been developed to measure rehabilitation outcomes, such as improved functional performance, increased independence, and enhanced quality of life.[29] Although many tools exist, a relatively small number of these are used frequently, with the most popular measures being range of movement, manual muscle testing, and Functional Independence Measure (FIM).[29] Many of these tools are not useful in the evaluation of AT as they do not allow the role of AT to be acknowledged in achieving rehabilitation outcomes.[13]

Increasingly, there are multiple stakeholders with an interest in evaluating the effectiveness of interventions such as AT, namely AT users and their significant others, individual service providers, service managers, funding bodies, and policy makers.[33,40] Evaluations may include one or multiple perspectives.[40] It is, therefore, important to understand the values and perspectives of each stakeholder and to balance these when choosing and interpreting outcomes.[80] Although some maintain that each of these stakeholders has a varying interest in the information they seek when evaluating interventions and services,[21,33] studies have yet to definitively support this contention.[33] Service managers and funding bodies are purported to have an active interest in the cost benefits of products or intervention approaches, whereas researchers and product developers are believed to be interested in the overall effectiveness of products or services.[54] Service providers and consumers, on the other hand, are thought to be more interested in the benefits of a particular device in a specific application.[54] However, consumers are becoming increasingly informed and interested in understanding the relative benefits of devices,[73] including cost benefits and the purported outcomes of interventions.[41] Different stakeholders may have different reasons for seeking information and deal with data in different ways, but all are concerned with establishing the benefits and identifying the associated costs of technology and services. Whether these stakeholders are examining information at an individual level to measure changes following an intervention or service, or aggregating data to determine the benefits of a range of products or service, essentially they all require information about the outcomes achieved by individuals or groups of consumers. The best way to evaluate the effectiveness of AT and associated services is to establish whether they meet the needs of the users.[4,36]

$$\text{Product/Program Effectiveness} = \frac{\text{Number of } \textit{Enabled} \text{ and } \textit{Satisfied} \text{ Consumers}}{\text{Total Number of Consumers}}$$

Outcome measurements must first examine the benefit of solutions for each consumer to establish the overall effectiveness of a product or service. Once the benefit of solutions for each individual has been established, these data can then be collated and analyzed to determine the overall effectiveness of services, products, or funding in meeting consumer need. Using consumer-centered outcome measures ensures that services, funding, and product design are consumer centered.

Given the diversity of technologies and AT users, this undertaking may seem overwhelming. However, many industries with multiple stakeholders have varying interests and a diverse consumer base with a range of expectations. Let's revisit our computer/car purchase from Chapter 3. It would not be unreasonable to expect that computer and car manufacturers have a very good understanding of their broad consumer base. These companies would know the demographics of their consumers, their expectations of products, the images they aspire to, what they want to use the products for, and where and how the product is to be used. They study the efficiency of the performance of their products in laboratories and in the field, and know the lifespan of every component and the impact of a range of climatic conditions. Market research provides them with information on whether their products meet consumer expectations and report on any difficulties the consumers experience in using the product. They know when people replace or upgrade their cars/computers, what information people need about new models, and what kind of products and services satisfy customer expectations. Commercial enterprises also have a very sound understanding of how to inform their consumer base about their products and services and what is required to support them with decision making.

Within a highly competitive commercial environment, these companies are acutely aware that they have to provide a quality product and associated services at a price that is acceptable to the consumer, the institutions that finance the purchase, and the government bodies that dictate safety requirements. Similarly, the AT industry requires a deep understanding of their consumers, their goals, expectations, and experiences to evaluate products and services and to establish an understanding of the range of outcomes that need to be examined. AT companies are becoming more aware of the value of understanding the diversity of AT users' preferences and needs, but to date have not systematically obtained user feedback about the effectiveness of their products.[72] AT users are ultimately in the best position to evaluate the effectiveness of these technologies.[4] This information can then, in turn, be used to inform their product development. People who have used technologies over an extended period are also in a good position to define the factors that need to be considered in developing evaluation criteria. Although consumer research may be considered by some to be a luxury that addresses consumer wants rather than needs, it is, in fact, essential to developing useful products, effective services, and good outcomes.[74,82]

The stakes are often high for people with disabilities when selecting a device. An inappropriate purchase is not just a financial burden; it can significantly affect health, restrict activity participation, and reduce quality of life. In addition, it is often difficult for people with disabilities to identify suitable technologies, as they are not always certain of their requirements, aware of what is possible, familiar with what is available, or able to access appropriate resources to explore and fund options. They often have complex needs where solutions are not readily identifiable or available. It is important that products are designed to meet *real* consumer need, and that the services are refined to ensure people with disabilities are afforded the best possible information and support. This is achieved with a better understanding of consumers, their goals and expectations, and their experiences of selecting and using technology. A better understanding of AT users and their experience of technology use is also fundemental to defining quality outcomes and identifying factors that contribute or detract from achieving these.

CONSUMER-CENTERED OUTCOME MEASUREMENT

A consumer-centered approach identifies and ensures that the user's needs are met. Traditionally, assistive technology providers (ATPs) have been concerned with the ability of a device to perform a specific function (e.g., move through space or input into a computer). Consumer-centered services then sought to ensure the device had the appropriate specifications for the user's dimensions and loss of function and that the user could operate the device. The importance of consumer preferences was not always acknowledged, and consumers were rarely afforded opportunities to choose between options in which the relative appearance and functions could be traded off between devices. More recently, a deeper understanding of the user's perceptions of technology has resulted in consumers being afforded the power to determine which aspects of the technology have greater importance for them and to choose a device (or other form of support) using these criteria. Service providers are also more sensitive to consumers' right to define their requirements and preferences and to determine if technology enables them to participate equitably in their activities of choice.

Although traditional practice placed emphasis on establishing the person's clinical status as defined and evaluated by the service provider,[50] consumer-centered practice encourages clients to choose and define outcomes that are meaningful to them. If we say we subscribe to consumer-centered practice, then the outcomes used to evaluate products and services must be meaningful to consumers[50] and reflect an understanding of the factors that affect consumer outcomes. Evaluation tools and processes should also be clearly linked to the purposes identified by the user.[74] The development of client-centered outcome measures requires an understanding of the following:

- The consumer's experience of selecting and using solutions and *why* outcome measurement may be useful to *consumers*
- The process consumers go through when selecting and using a solution and *when* outcome measurement is required
- Things that are important to consumers in the process of selecting and using solutions and *what* outcomes need to be measured
- Information required by consumers to direct the process and *how* outcomes are best determined and presented

UTILITY OF OUTCOME MEASUREMENT FOR CONSUMERS

From the consumer's perspective, consumer-centered outcome measurement ensures that outcomes of value to the consumer are identified and used in such a way that consumers have control of the process and are provided with a deeper understanding of their needs and requirements so that they are better able to manage their AT needs in the long term. Consumer-centered outcomes provide a structure for collaboration and transparent decision-making, which allows consumers to do the following:

- Identify and articulate their goals and preferences, in order to shape the process
- Determine the criteria on which solutions are evaluated
- Understand the strengths and limitations of each solution

- Present evidence of the benefits of the proposed solution to the funding body in the way in which they want them presented, emphasizing participation rather than dysfunction
- Determine if the solution is working as expected in the application environment and if not, examine what is impacting on the solution
- Understand the impact of the solution on their comfort and participation
- Examine whether the solution is meeting changing requirements (e.g., user expectations and skill, change in task demands)
- Monitor the ongoing effectiveness of the solution and its capacity to respond to changes in context
- Determine when a solution is no longer meeting expectations

▇ WHEN SHOULD OUTCOMES BE EVALUATED?

When examining the experiences of AT users throughout the process of selecting and using technology in the workplace, it is evident that there are distinct steps in the process (Box 9-1). Each stage of the process attends to different aspects of the AT system and, therefore, requires focused evaluation.[103] The overall evaluation of the process and outcome would be the culmination of the outcomes at each stage.[103] The long-term success of the technology is dependent on quality outcomes at each step in the process. For example, without clearly defining the goals and specifying the requirements of the device, the exploration of technology can lack focus and the selected device may not ultimately meet the user's requirements. Equally, the quality of outcomes at each step in the process is dependent on a sound understanding of the whole process and the long-term

---

BOX 9-1
Steps in the Process of Selecting and Using Technology

1. Visioning possibilities
2. Establishing goals/expectations
3. Identifying specific requirements
4. Defining required features
5. Obtaining information on potential technologies and resources
6. Locating local resources and supports
7. Developing a funding strategy
8. Trialing and evaluating options
9. Purchasing device
10. Integrating device with other technologies
11. Customizing device to personal requirements
12. Mastering use of the device
13. Maintaining and repairing the device
14. Insuring the device
15. Reviewing ongoing suitability
16. Upgrading the technology as the need arises

expectations of the technology. If adequate consideration is not given to the flexibility and adjustability required of the technology in the workplace, the chosen device may not be able to respond to the inevitable changes in the user's skill, work tasks, or the work environment.

The experiences of AT users have highlighted factors that contributed to the success of each step in the process and that contribute to or limit the effective long-term use of the technology. These experiences suggest outcomes to be expected at each step, which ensure the user is able to progress to the next step and which also contribute to the quality of the final outcome. Each step of the process enables consumers to develop a deeper understanding of their requirements and the resources available to assist them in identifying and acquiring their technology. In addition, each step contributes to a clearer understanding of the requirements of the technology. The expected outcomes for the consumer and the technology at each step are outlined in Table 9-1.

The selection and use of assistive technology is also cyclical, in that each stage offers a deeper understanding of the requirements and expectations of the technology.[103] Experience with technology results in the user developing skills and a better understanding of how technology might be used.[48] It is important that changes in requirements and expectations are tracked throughout the process. It is not assumed that the user has the same understandings and expectations at the end of the process that they have at the beginning of the process. A number of the AT users in this study lamented that they wished they had the benefit of experience before embarking on the process. Those with prior experience of technology reported feeling better placed to anticipate their needs and detail the requirements of the technology. Experienced services providers often were able to assist inexperienced users to realize their needs and define their goals but were not always able to predict issues that may arise for the user when using the device over the long term. For many AT users, the process extends well beyond their contact with service providers who primarily assist with the selection and acquisition of technology. Consumers faced many challenges in implementing technology in the application environment, adapting the solution to their changing requirements, and dealing with numerous demands placed on the solution as things changed over time. Equipping consumers to understand and manage these issues is an important part of the process.

Users will go through the process of investigation and AT integration repeatedly throughout their working life. Rather than being a "one-time, all-or-nothing proposition" (p. 8),[53] it is a decision-making process that recurs over time.[53] Although services are currently focused on evaluating the suitability of the technology in meeting the user's immediate needs, outcome measurement also should be extended to assess the ongoing suitability of the solution. AT users need to be able periodically to review their technology to ensure it is still meeting their needs. Changes in skills and abilities, the nature of work tasks, the platform technologies, and demands in the work environment can often mean that the technology is no longer suitable and may need further adjustment or replacement. Developing a capacity to evaluate the ongoing suitability of

TABLE 9-1

Expected Outcomes for Each Step in the Process of Technology Selection and Use

STEPS IN THE PROCESS	EXPECTED CONSUMER OUTCOMES	EXPECTED TECHNOLOGY OUTCOMES
Visioning possibilities	Willingness to explore technology Aware of what is technologically possible Aware of technologic developments	Technology in use Technology is most up-to-date solution available for the purpose
Establishing goals/expectations	Clearly identified goals	Solution meets goals
Identifying specific requirements	Details of person, task, technology, and environment requirements identified Consumer aware of preferences Requirements account for future needs	Solution meets preferences Meets current requirements—person task environment Meets future requirements
Defining required features	Specifications for technology listed Aware of range of options	
Obtaining information on potential technologies and resources	Consumer directs decision making	
Locating local resources and supports	Comprehensive list of local resources compiled, including other users User accesses local resources and supports	
Developing a funding strategy	Funding does not place restrictions on device type or use	Funding covers preferred device and associated costs Preferred solution identified
Trialing and evaluating options	Suitable options trialed in situ User has understanding of strengths and limitations of each option User confident with choice	
Purchasing device	Device procured in timely manner User is satisfied with funding and acquisition process	Preferred device purchased
Integrating device into the workplace	User able to participate equitably in workplace User feels accepted and valued Employer and co-workers aware of specific requirements of technologies	Technology set up in timely manner Technology working consistently in context Device is accepted and managed in the workplace
Customizing device to personal requirements	User can adjust device to meet personal requirements	Device is adjusted to provide comfortable and efficient use throughout the day

TABLE 9-1

(cont'd)

STEPS IN THE PROCESS	EXPECTED CONSUMER OUTCOMES	EXPECTED TECHNOLOGY OUTCOMES
Mastering use of the device	User does not experience any discomfort or strain User understands features of the device User has adequate time to learn to use device and develop confidence User can operate device confidently User able to access suitable training support in a timely manner (i.e., as required)	Device is easy to learn and use Device provides adequate manual, help screen, or online support
Maintaining and repairing the device	User has access to backup technology User has timely access to IT/manufacturer support	Device in good working order Minimum technological error/down time
Insuring the device	Device can be replaced if not functional	
Reviewing ongoing suitability	User can identify changing needs Process established in workplace for periodic review User has access to appropriate supports for reviewing and identifying needs and initiating requests User and employer are satisfied with work productivity Employer and co-workers aware of need for periodic review Employer aware of resources to access when reviewing technology requirements Employer notifies user of impending changes in the workplace	Device allows full participation in the workplace Device can be adjusted to meet changing needs Device can be used across activities and settings including home
Upgrading the technology as the need arises	User can identify when solution no longer meets his/her needs Employer accesses appropriate resources when upgrading technology User is informed when upgrades of the device are available	Device is updated and supported as needed

equipment is critical to the long-term viability of the user in the workplace. The ultimate outcome for any technology solution is that the user has *ready* access to their *preferred* technology and that it is *reliable,* enables them to carry out their preferred *activities* with *ease* and *efficiency* in both the *short* and *long* term within all the required *contexts.*

WHAT TO EVALUATE

Typically, "what gets measured gets managed" (p. 101).[12] If we are to manage the process of selecting and using technology effectively, then we need to ensure we are measuring the *right* outcomes. Deciding on which outcomes to measure and how to measure them is among the most problematic aspects of evaluation.[21,33] Outcomes are a multidimensional concept that can include user satisfaction, functional independence, increased social participation, enhanced normative social roles, the promotion and sustaining of employment, and facilitation of activities of daily living.[38] The nature of the outcomes measured is determined by a number of factors, namely, the conceptual model the evaluator is operating from and the nature of measures available. Some propose that the future of effective outcome measurement is dependent on theories about the adoption of AT being developed.[35,53,79] A solid theoretical foundation would assist the industry in defining the expected outcomes of AT interventions, identify factors that affect AT outcomes, and develop suitable outcome measures. It is important to be aware of the theoretical framework guiding evaluation and the conceptualizations that are defining the factors being examined and shaping the choice of measures. It is equally important to review the tools available and determine how well these align with our understanding and acknowledge areas of evaluation that are not being adequately addressed by these measures.

To date, outcomes measurement has lacked explicit theorization.[33] Without an adequate theoretical foundation, service providers use a haphazard approach to evaluation[52,53] and find it difficult to select appropriate outcome measures and provide an adequate explanation for the findings.[33] Traditionally, products and services have been developed with use of a rehabilitation frame of reference and, as such, have focused on designing products that replace lost function, allocating devices according to diagnosis or nature and level of impairment and then fitting the device to the disability. Outcomes in this model have tended to focus on clinical results, functional status, and objective indicators of quality of life.[22] The tools developed within this model measure performance of the individual against established "norms." These measures are often taken immediately after the intervention in an effort to establish its efficacy and are often viewed as being stable beyond the point of measurement.

More recently, evaluation has been driven by policymakers and payers,[22] which has resulted in an emphasis on the cost effectiveness of products and services rather than on clinical outcomes.[20,40] There has been a sustained interest in AT use and nonuse and the cost benefits of AT over interventions requiring ongoing expenditure, such as personal assistants. However, investigation has been limited to consumer dissatisfaction with devices they are forced to use in the absence of more suitable alternatives or the underuse of potentially effective devices.[33] There is a great need for a better understanding of why some devices are more effective than others for particular people to achieve specific goals and in certain environments.

Effective measurement requires a systematic approach to identifying and defining suitable outcomes. The AT field has been seeking a suitable model for practice and outcomes measurement that is both descriptive and predictive.[52,53] Although no theory has dominated,[52] a number of theories have provided a rich description of the AT system and factors that impact effective device use, such as the Human, Activity and Assistive Technology (HAAT)[13] and Matching Person and Technology (MPT)[84,85] models. These models seek to explain the complex interaction between the technology and the person, the goals or activities to be undertaken, and the environment.

More recently, there have been attempts to develop predictive models that identify expected outcomes. Fuhrer,[35] Lenker and Paquet,[53] and Smith[91] have independently drawn on existing AT practice models, parallel interventions models,[93] social cognitive, and perceived attributes theories[77] to provide a schema for predicting AT use and outcomes. Although it is not the intention to provide a review of these models in this text, there are elements in these models that bear noting. Each of these models outlines a causal pathway from the point of procurement, which identifies contextual factors that impact on AT outcomes and recognizes the role of the person, task, and environment in determining the suitability of AT and how these influence the ongoing use of technology. Because assistive devices are likely to be one of a number of possible interventions, such as the use of personal assistance, the use of AT is weighed against the benefits of alternative interventions.[89] Effective device use may also be linked with other interventions, such as redesigning of the activity or the environment being undertaken simultaneously. An AT outcome system needs to understand and document baseline function[89] and the outcomes the user seeks from an AT intervention.[33,89] The AT process is also recognized as being cyclical with intention to use AT being continuously reevaluated.[53] AT use also needs to be considered from both short- and long-term vantage points,[35] as it not possible to reliably predict long-term use based solely on an initial trial period. The perceived benefits of AT use are identified in these models as being subjective well-being,[35] quality of life,[53] as well as enhanced function,[89] effectiveness, efficiency, and device satisfaction[35] or usability.[53] Continued AT use is identified as the primary indicator of success in both the Fuhrer[35] and Lenker and Paquet[53] outcome frameworks, whereas Smith's IMPACT 2 model identifies enhanced function as the primary outcome of AT use.[89] It is very difficult to capture the complex interactions between these variables and the impact of these and other factors on AT use. However, each of these authors strives to provide a better understanding of AT use, the factors affecting use, and outcomes that result from using AT.

▣ DOMAINS OF EVALUATION

A number of domains have been commonly associated with AT outcome measurement, namely device usability, user satisfaction, quality of life, social role performance, functional level, and cost.[54] Broadly, outcomes can be conceptualized at three levels: personal, AT system, and service delivery. Personal outcomes relate to the well-being, sense of accomplishment, and experience of life resulting from the use of AT. AT system outcomes address the consequences of the fit between the technology and the person, tasks, and environment, the user's experience of the device, and the process. Service outcomes investigate the impact of AT in general, and examine device use, the cost-utility of devices, and their effect on participation. Interest in these domains has resulted in a number of tools being developed specifically for the evaluation of AT; however, more generic tools have also been used in the evaluation of AT.

Assistive Technology System Outcomes

The HAAT model,[13] which focuses on "someone, doing something, somewhere" provides a useful foundation for evaluating the effectiveness of an AT system. It does not have an assessment form and is intended to provide a framework within which the AT system is seen as dynamic, where changes are anticipated in the person's goals and abilities, tasks, AT, or the environment (see Figure 2-1). The effectiveness of the AT system is determined by measuring the performance of the AT system; that is, the ability of the person to successfully complete activities using the AT in the application environments. This model proposes that the effectiveness of AT is measured by evaluating the performance of the AT *system*, that is, the interaction between the human, the activities being performed, the AT used, and the environment in which it is performed. Consequently, outcomes measurement focuses on how well a device works, for whom, doing what, and under which real-life circumstances.[33] A good AT solution is a good *fit* between the technology and the person, the technology and the activities being undertaken, the technology and other devices, and between the technology and the environment. Outcome measurement should focus on determining how well the AT interacts with the person, the activities and tasks, and the context (Figure 9-1).

A range of parameters has been identified in the literature as being important considerations when evaluating the effectiveness of technology. When examining the fit between the person and the technology (Figure 9-2), the effectiveness of the device would be determined by establishing how well the device meets the goals of the person[85] and matches the skills and abilities of the person.[85,95] The device also should be easy to use and operate.[4,103] The person's satisfaction with the appearance[4,95,103] and his overall satisfaction would also need to be evaluated.[18,19,95,100] The device would need to increase the user's sense of competence, confidence, and independence.[16] The person would also need to feel comfortable[4,95,103] when using it, and use it with minimal effort for appropriate periods.[95] If required, the device should be portable.[4] It should not expose the person to any risk of injury and should be able to be customized and adjusted to meet the person's specific daily requirements[4,95,103] and long-term

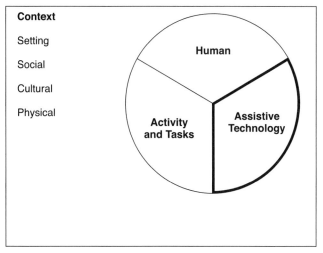

FIGURE 9-1 ▦ Interaction between the AT and the human, activity, and environment

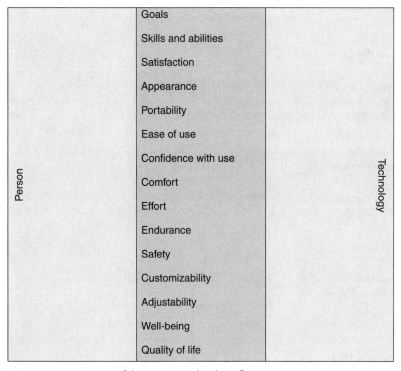

FIGURE 9-2 ▦ Outcome of the person-technology fit.

needs. The device should promote the user's well-being[16] and assist the user in achieving an acceptable quality of life.[43,44]

A good fit between the technology and the activity (Figure 9-3) should result in the device being used consistently to complete intended tasks.[53,103] The usability of the device would be reflected in the person feeling productive[16] and able to undertake these tasks efficiently[16] and effectively.[53] The device should also enable the person to move between and complete the required range of tasks effectively.[4] The device should also be dependable or in working order at all times.[4,95]

The degree to which the device fits with the environment(s) (Figure 9-4) requires that the device is affordable in the first instance[4,95] with ongoing costs being acceptable and manageable.[2,103] The device would need to be easily assembled and maintained[4,103] in the environment and adequately secured to prevent displacement or theft.[4] It should be accessible to the user whenever and wherever it is needed.[95] The device would also need to present an image that is acceptable to others, appropriate for the application environment,[4,95,103] and compatible with furnishings, other technologies, and people within the en-

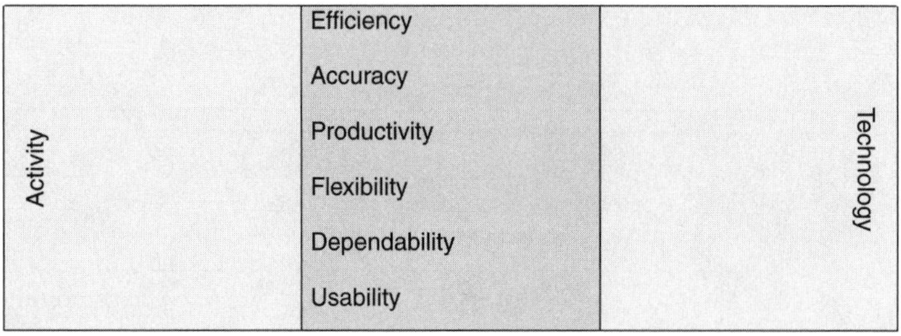

Activity	Efficiency	Technology
	Accuracy	
	Productivity	
	Flexibility	
	Dependability	
	Usability	

FIGURE 9-3 ■ Outcomes of the activity-technology fit.

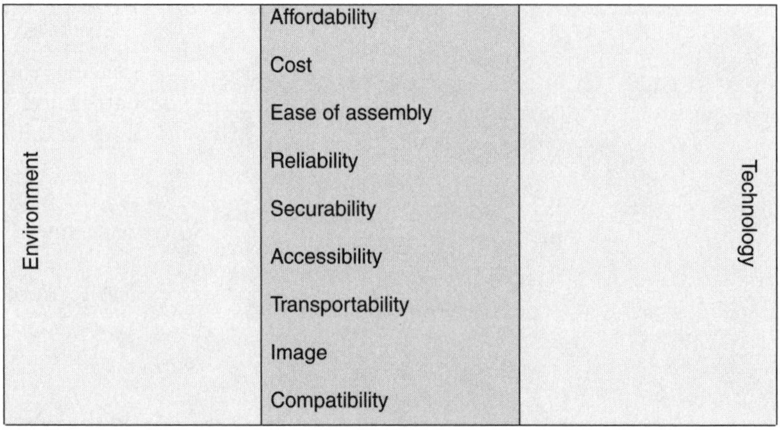

Environment	Affordability	Technology
	Cost	
	Ease of assembly	
	Reliability	
	Securability	
	Accessibility	
	Transportability	
	Image	
	Compatibility	

FIGURE 9-4 ■ Outcome of the person-environment fit.

vironment.[4,103] The device should be durable and able to withstand the demands of the environment.[4]

AT System outcomes evaluation examines the degree of fit between the following:

- Person and AT: goals, satisfaction, skills and abilities, efficacy, and impact (fatigue and pain)
- AT and activity: effective and efficient performance of relevant tasks
- AT and other devices: technical performance, support required, and longevity/upgradeability
- AT and the environments (physical, cultural, social): across environments, perception of others, impact on/from environment, and degree to which it fits with cultural values and beliefs

The fit needs to be evaluated repeatedly throughout the process as goals and expectations develop and requirements become evident. Furthermore, the fit requires ongoing evaluation in order to assess the impact of changes in the person's skills and abilities, task requirements, and environmental demands.

A range of tools has been developed to address a variety of parameters identified above; however, some parameters are not examined by existing outcome measures. Evaluation of fit requires a mixture of objective and qualitative measures that allow for the uniqueness of each system and quality of performance to be examined. Although a number of self-report measures have been developed, few objective measures examine fit.[52]

Personal Outcomes

Assistive devices enable people to be more independent and take advantage of life's possibilities.[43,63] It is vital that consumers are provided with mechanisms to evaluate and compare solutions against their identified goals, preferences, and requirements. It is important to note that the success of the outcome is also dependent on *how well* goals, preferences, and requirements are established in the first instance.[87] Although some AT users are very clear about their goals, preferences, and requirements when seeking an AT intervention, others require structure and support to be able to articulate these clearly. A number of tools have been developed that provide a structure for developing goals and identifying preferences and requirements, as well as a means of evaluating how well devices meet these. The assessment instruments from the MPT[85] process examines the person's perceptions of strengths and capabilities, needs/goals, preferences, and psychosocial characteristics, as well as expectations regarding the benefits of technology. The Assistive Technology Device Predisposition Assessment[85] is the measure that focuses on personal technologies designed to enhance an individual's functioning, whereas the items on the Workplace Technology Predisposition Assessment (WT PA)[85] identify barriers or enhancements to the use of more generalized products used by employees. The WT PA examines the employee's and employer's expectations of technology considered to most likely affect AT use (Figure 9-5). Although originally designed to assist in the selection process, these tools also have been used to evaluate the effectiveness of

A

Employee Name _____   Date _____

Technology _____

Employees who feel threatened or uncomfortable with new technology cannot use that technology in a manner beneficial to themselves, the company or institution. This survey will assist you in identifying areas that could affect your acceptance or use of a new technology in the workplace. This form should be used together with the companion *Employer Form*

The Technology Itself	*Definitely*		*Somewhat*		*Not at All*
Is the technology useable with little or no discomfort, stress, or fatigue?	5	4	3	2	1
Is the length of time needed for training reasonable?	5	4	3	2	1
Is this technology different from what you are currently using to accomplish the task?	5	4	3	2	1
Do you think mastering the technology will help you succeed?	5	4	3	2	1
Do you think mastering the technology will help you in the eyes of your peers and supervisors?	5	4	3	2	1

The Person Being Trained to Use the Technology	*Definitely*		*Somewhat*		*Not at All*
Have you had previous success with new technology in the work enviroment?	5	4	3	2	1
Are you generally in support of bringing a new technology into the workplace?	5	4	3	2	1
Do you feel you have a choice in how quickly the new technology will be installed?	5	4	3	2	1
Do you think you have the skills needed to use the new technology?	5	4	3	2	1
Do you feel that you fit in and belong in this workplace?	5	4	3	2	1
Are you satisfied with your current job?	5	4	3	2	1
Do you have what you need to do your job effectively?	5	4	3	2	1
Are your relationships with co-workers generally positive?	5	4	3	2	1
Are your relationships with your supervisor /employer generally positive?	5	4	3	2	1
Are you often working at or above your capacity level?	5	4	3	2	1
Do you feel expectations held by your employer are realistic?	5	4	3	2	1

FIGURE 9-5 ■ Workplace Technology Predisposition Assessment (WT PA). **A**, An instrument for employees, students, and others learning a new technology; **B**, An instrument for employers, trainers, and office managers.

The Milieu or Workplace Environment

	Definitely		Somewhat		Not at All
Do you have the level of support you want from your employer?	5	4	3	2	1
Do you believe there are enough promotional opportunities for you?	5	4	3	2	1
Do you believe your employer is open to the use of AT and other supports?	5	4	3	2	1
Is there an appropriate degree of teamwork at this worksite?	5	4	3	2	1
Do you feel employees' efforts are respected and appreciated in your office?	5	4	3	2	1
Will your AT use be independent of cooperation /assistance from co-workers and others who may feel inconvenienced by it?	5	4	3	2	1
Has sufficient time been allotted for training you in the new technology?	5	4	3	2	1
Have the benefits of the new technology been made clear to you?	5	4	3	2	1
Have training plans taken into consideration your learning style?	5	4	3	2	1
Do you feel you will be rewarded for mastering this technology?	5	4	3	2	1
Does the training occur where you can become familiar with the new technology and make mistakes in a non-threatening atmosphere?	5	4	3	2	1

How Well Does Everything Match?

Employers (or trainers) and employee(s) should discuss the responses to items on this form and the companion employer form. Plans should be developed to address those issues that received a negative rating. Discrepancies between employer and employee on the various concepts should be discussed. The space below can be used to list and address the most important of these discrepancies and negative influences.

Discrepancy or Negative Influence	Plan for Addressing Discrepancy or Issue
_____	_____
_____	_____
_____	_____
_____	_____

COMMENTS AND NOTES:

FIGURE 9-5 (*cont'd*)

B

Employee Name _____ Date _____

Technology _____

Employees who feel threatened or uncomfortable with new technology cannot use that technology in a manner beneficial to the company or institution. This instrument will assist you in identifying areas which could inhibit the acceptance or appropriate use ot a new technology within the work environment. This form should be used in conjunction with the companion Employee Form.

The Technology Itself

	Positive Influence		Neutral Influence		Negative Influence
Is the technology useable with little or no discomfort, stress, or fatigue?	5	4	3	2	1
Is the length of time needed for training a positive or negative aspect of acceptance?	5	4	3	2	1
How different is the technology from what is currently being used by the employee(s)?	5	4	3	2	1
Can the technology be introduced into the workplace gradually or must it be accepted all at once?	5	4	3	2	1
Does mastering the technology confer status to the user?	5	4	3	2	1

The Person(s) Being Trained to Use the Technology

	Positive		Neutral		Negative
Has the employee(s) had previous success with new technologies in the work environment?	5	4	3	2	1
Is the employee(s) generally in support of bringing the new technology into the workplace?	5	4	3	2	1
Does the employee(s) feel they have a choice in how quickly the new technology will be installed?	5	4	3	2	1
Does the employee(s) possess the skills needed to use the new technology?	5	4	3	2	1
Does the employee(s) know how he/she best learns the use of such new technologies (e.g., instructions given individually, in groups, in writing, verbally, etc.)	5	4	3	2	1

The Milieu or Workplace Environment

	Positive		Neutral		Negative
Does the employee(s) feel his/her efforts are respected and appreciated?	5	4	3	2	1

FIGURE 9-5 (*cont'd*)

| Has sufficient time been allotted for training in the new technology? | 5 | 4 | 3 | 2 | 1 |

| Have the benefits of the new technology been made clear to all employees? | 5 | 4 | 3 | 2 | 1 |

| Have training plans taken into consideration the varying learning styles of individual employees? | 5 | 4 | 3 | 2 | 1 |

| Will the employee(s) be rewarded for mastering the new technology? | 5 | 4 | 3 | 2 | 1 |

| Does the training provide an atmosphere where the employee(s) can become familiar with the new technology and make mistakes in a non-threatening atmosphere? | 5 | 4 | 3 | 2 | 1 |

How Well Does Everything Match?

Many (perhaps even most) of the situations where individuals encounter technology contain some element of choice. For example, we may be required to stand in line for a long time, but we can still refuse to use ATMs. We can reject cordless telephones, microwave ovens and VCRs. However the workplace is often the one environment where such a choice is denied us. Frequently, decisions concerning the adoption and use of such technologies are made, not by the users, but by their supervisors. Time spent by the employees and the trainers considering the concepts on this form will lead to more effective adaptation and use of expensive technology.

Employers (or trainers) and the employee(s) being trained should discuss their responses to items on this form. Plans should be developed to address those issues that received a negative influence rating from both of you. Any discrepancies between employer and employee on the various concepts should be discussed. The space below can be used to list and address the most important of these discrepancies and negative influences.

Discrepancy or Negative Influence	Plan for Addressing Discrepancy or Issue
_____	_____
_____	_____
_____	_____
_____	_____

FIGURE 9-5 (*cont'd*)

technology interventions and have demonstrated some ability to predict outcomes.[83] In addition, rehabilitation counselors trained in the MPT model and using a consumer-driven process for device selection achieved "enhanced AT service delivery outcomes" (p. 1321)[85]; that is, the employees assisted by trained providers continued to use the devices that were purchased.

The Canadian Occupational Performance Measure (COPM)[51] is an individualized evaluation tool that uses a semistructured interview to help consumers identify specific problems in occupational performance areas, such as self-care, productivity, and leisure.[17] The importance of each problem is then rated on a scale of 1 (not important) to 10 (very important). Next, the client rates their current level of performance and satisfaction on scales of 1 (unable to perform, not satisfied) to 10 (able to perform, extremely satisfied). This, in turn, can impact their quality of life and sense of well-being. While not designed to address assistive technology devices specifically, this tool allows the client to reassess his or her performance on the identified tasks at various intervals, evaluate the change resulting from an intervention, and determine if there is any change in performance in the longer term. In a recent review of the use of the COPM as an outcome measure, Carswell et al. found the COPM had been used with a variety of client groups in practice and outcomes research over the last decade.[11] More specifically, it has been used in a number of studies to determine the impact of rehabilitation[28,90] and assistive devices,[6,11,67,97] and was found to be sensitive to changes that result from these interventions[11] and able to provide information that cannot be obtained from less individualized measures.[17]

A recent review of rehabilitation providers in Europe and Australia found a great diversity in the range of outcome measures used by rehabilitation providers, with most interest focused on changes in physical status rather than quality-of-life outcomes.[29,39] Despite the availability of numerous quality of life measures,[65] measuring quality-of-life outcomes is more common in the research community than in rehabilitation services.[29,39] This could be because quality of life is a general outcome, which may not be attributable to a specific intervention outside a controlled research context. In an effort to capture the impact of an assistive device on the user's competence, self-esteem, and adaptability, Day and Jutai designed the Psychosocial Impact of Assistive Devices Scale (PIADS).[16] The PIADS is a 26-item self-report questionnaire that requires AT users to indicate the impact of a specific AT device on items that reflect important psychosocial constructs in evaluating AT devices. The three subscales are (1) competence, (2) self-esteem, and (3) adaptability. The AT user is asked to rate the degree to which the device decreases (-3) or increases (+3) their competence, happiness, independence, adequacy, confusion, efficiency, self-esteem, productivity, security, frustration, usefulness, self-confidence, expertise, skillfulness, well-being, capability, quality of life, performance, sense of power, sense of control, embarrassment, willingness to take chances, eagerness to try new things, and ability to participate, adapt to activities of daily living, and take advantage of opportunities. The PIADS has been used to evaluate a range of assistive devices, such as eyeglasses and contact lenses,[16,45] closed circuit televisions,[96] electronic daily living aids,[46] powered mobility devices,[9] and hearing aids.[81] This tool has been well constructed and is psychometrically sound.[33] However, some users may find some of the items difficult to differentiate and respond to. For example, some people may not be able to distinguish between sense of control and sense of power and may not feel that a device affects them in this way. The tool also is better suited to evaluating the impact of a device after a period of use rather than providing a structure for comparing devices following a short-term trial. Further exploration also would be required to determine why a device may increase or decrease productivity or feelings of confusion.

The Individualized Prioritized Problem Assessment (IPPA)[102] is a similar tool that was specifically designed to assess the impact of assistive devices. Through an interview, this tool allows clients to identify problems and to rate the importance and degree of difficulty the person experiences in carrying out the activity on a FIM-like 7-point scale, with 1 being of no importance at all, not at all difficult, and 7 being most important, too difficult to perform activity. This tool provides a list of daily activities similar to many chapter or first-level activities listed in the International Classification of Functioning, Disability, and Health (ICF),[106] namely self-care, mobility, transportation, housework, safety, leisure, communication, work, and social interaction, as a foundation for discussing potential problems with AT users. It enables issues to be prioritized and the baseline performance to then be compared with performance following acquisition of the device.[102] The IPPA also asks the AT user to rate on a 5-point scale how the AT has addressed each problem, with -2 being much less than expected and +2 being much more than expected. This tool has not been used extensively in outcome studies but was found in one study to be a useful individualized measure for evaluating AT device and service delivery outcomes.[101]

Another tool that has been used in rehabilitation research and offers promise in the area of evaluating AT outcomes is the Goal Attainment Scale (GAS).[102] Originally designed for use in community mental health settings, this tool allows individualized goals to be established and outcomes to be defined in clear behavioral terms.[27] Typically, outcomes are developed for each goal on a 5-point scale, with 0 being the most likely outcome, +2 being the most favorable outcome and -2 being the least favorable outcome.[57] GAS has a protocol for developing the goal outcomes that must be strictly adhered to.[27] This protocol requires that the goal setter and assessor be independent of the service provider who provides the intervention. To date, studies suggest that GAS is a clinically useful and responsive tool for measuring rehabilitation and AT outcomes.[78,88] However, developing suitable scales for each goal requires training and experience.[88] The complexity of the tool is reflected in the fact that few studies adhere to the structure and protocol provided.[27]

User Satisfaction

Consumers' level of satisfaction with the solution and their perception of whether their goals, preferences, and requirements have been met are important when examining their perceptions of the effectiveness of service and the success of the solution. Some measures of satisfaction seek a global judgment of satisfaction from the user, whereas others examine specific characteristics of the device.[54] Global measures of user satisfaction are typically positively skewed[52]; however, this bias can be mitigated when items probe for satisfaction with specific elements of products or services.[47] The Quebec User Evaluation of Satisfaction with assistive Technology (QUEST)[18] is a 12-item outcome measure that was designed specifically to evaluate user satisfaction with assistive devices (eight items) and services (four items).[19] This tool recognizes that satisfaction is a multidimensional concept that is influenced by the user's expectations, perceptions, attitudes, and values.[19] AT users are asked to rate their satisfaction with the device and services on a 5-point scale, with 1 being not satisfied at all and 5 being very satisfied. The device is rated according to its weight, comfort, durability, adjustments, simplicity of use, dimensions, effectiveness, and safety, and the service is rated in terms of delivery, professional service, follow-up, and repairs and servicing. Space is also provided for comment on each item. Users are then asked to indicate the three most important items for the device from the 12 items provided. This tool has been used in research and clinically and is currently available in seven languages. It has been found to be useful when evaluating user satisfaction with a range of AT such as mobility, bathing devices, and switch toys.[5] It is also establishing itself as a reliable and valid outcome measure in research studies, with more studies expected to be published in the near future.[19]

User satisfaction is an important aspect of outcome measurement, and self-administered questionnaires are easy to use; however, concerns have been raised about the exclusive use of these tools.[33] First, satisfaction is closely linked to the persons' expectations. If the person has low expectations, then their satisfaction may be inflated, as compared with someone with high expectations. Expectations are also likely to change over time in response to marketing, information, or experience with the device, which would then result in differences in satisfaction depending on when the measure was taken.[33] Second, objective measures help ensure that more objective information is obtained regarding the functional performance of the device. Objective measures provide the user, service provider, and payer with information about the ability of the device to enhance function.

Usability

Evaluating the usability of products has been an important theme in the field of human computer interaction (HCI) for some time.[72] Usability is defined by the ISO 9241 Version 2.5 as "comprising the effectiveness, efficiency and satisfaction with which a user can achieve a specific goal within a particular environment."[52,72,103] Usability is not a property of the device per se,[54] but rather examines the fit between the technology and the person, the tasks, and environment. Indicators of usability include quality of task performance, error rates, ease of learning, effort, comfort, time required to complete the task, the quality of the end product, and satisfaction.[53,54,99] Both subjective and objective measures are required to examine usability.

Subjective measures allow the user to evaluate how well the device fits personal priorities, the tasks he or she performs, and the environments in which the tasks are performed, such as is done with the ATD PA and WTPA. Usability is an individual construct that can vary from person to person.[103] Evaluation tools can, therefore, be specifically selected to address aspects of the person, task, or environment interaction that are of particular importance to the person and the nature of the AT system being evaluated. For example, the user's perceptions of whether the device increases competence, self-esteem, and adaptability can be evaluated using the PIADS. Satisfaction with comfort, adjustments, simplicity of use, and effectiveness can be evaluated using the QUEST. Standardized self-report measures are also available that evaluate pain such as Verbal Rating Scales (VRS), Visual Analogue Scales (VASs), and Picture scales, as well as pain questionnaires.[66] Various tools have been constructed for clinical use that allow users to comment on or rate aspects of the fit using Likert scales and semantic differential scales. Although these tools may not be standardized, they provide the user and service providers with feedback on specific aspects of the AT system that are either working or not working for the individual.

Self-report data are essential in understanding the user's perception of the fit, but they may not provide an assessment of whether the AT system is being used optimally. For example, some users are unaware of what is causing their pain and may not attribute it to the AT system. Other users may not be aware of features of the device that could reduce errors and may be happy with their level of efficiency, not knowing that it could be improved.

Objective measures of performance or activity output can provide valuable information about the efficiency and effectiveness of a device. Measures of output and error rate can assist the user to compare devices and to monitor ongoing performance so that changes can be addressed. Information also can be gathered over time about the number of times repairs and maintenance are required and the length of time devices are out of action, so that benchmarks for time in use can be established for assistive devices. Detailed information about the performance or activity output can be obtained by using specialized tools, such as COMPASS.[49] This software measures the user's computer performance, recording text entry, mouse, or pointer use and information processing, and provides quantitative data regarding reaction time, typing speed, and number of errors. COMPASS is a dedicated assessment program, so performance in the real world is not the objective. In many cases, it would also be useful to be able to collect data continuously on task performance, such as error and input speed by having software running in the background on the computer.[54] This would allow users to review the usability of the device throughout the day to evaluate how well it was meeting their needs. Because usability is dynamic, in that it varies over time[103] and with fatigue, mood, etc., it is important that periodic evaluation is undertaken to determine if the technology is meeting changing requirements.

Clinical evaluation of performance can also be useful when evaluating the usability of technology. Service providers can map pressure areas or assess changes in tone and posture, which may have long-term implications. Service providers are skilled in the use of clinical tools and observations to identify potential problem areas. This information needs to be communicated to users in a meaningful way so that they are able to understand and act on the service provider's concerns. More objective documentation of issues and evidence of their impact on long-term use would provide users and payers with the information they require to respond to recommendations.

Societal Outcomes

Societal outcomes are the most complex of all outcomes to quantify but are the outcomes that are of interest to the greatest number of stakeholders.[40] Societal outcomes, such as AT use and cost benefits, assist stakeholders in determining the relative merits of various interventions.[40]

Assistive Technology Use

As noted previously, there are numerous studies, which have investigated AT use. Most of these studies have measured use dichotomously, that is, use versus nonuse or abandonment.[53] However, there are other dimensions of device use that require closer examination if we are to understand the quality of AT outcomes. Frequency and duration of use have been identified as being meaningful dimensions in evaluating the quality of AT use.[5,53,54] In addition, understanding when and where devices are used and which activities they are used for also provides insight into the usefulness of AT devices.[54] Similarly, when and where devices are not used and which activities they are not used for also will provide valuable information on the limitations of devices. To date these aspects of device use have not been routinely evaluated.

When examining nonuse, it is also important to establish the reasons. Nonuse may result from improvements in the user's condition such that the device is no longer necessary.[15,69,104] Alternatively, the device may not be meeting the user's needs adequately.[14,54] Although lack of consumer involvement in the process of device selection has been found to predict discontinued use of devices, relative advantage has been found to be the strongest predictor of AT use.[73] In the study undertaken by Reimer-Reiss and Wacker, relative advantage was determined by comparing the benefits of a device, such as dependability, operability, and effectiveness, with the costs of device use.[73] It is important, therefore, that the usability of devices is examined carefully and weighed against the ongoing costs if AT use is to be promoted.

Cost-Utility

When examining the cost of assistive devices, many services focus primarily on the purchase price. Although this might seem logical in determining whether a device is affordable, it often results in a distortion of the cost-outcome analysis.[1] Cost is an economic concept that refers to the use of resources rather than the exchange of monies.[40] Resources used can include direct and indirect costs, such as equipment, provider salaries, service costs, formal and informal support costs, lost work time, and travel.[40] In terms of the initial purchase price, a mouthstick is considerably cheaper than a voice recognition system; however, when factoring the additional social costs incurred over 10 years, for example working days lost due to neck pain, productivity, and longevity of working life, the voice recognition system would prove to be more cost effective. Cost-utility evaluations consider the nonmonetary outcomes rather than limiting analysis to only the monetary benefits of AT.[40]

In an effort to quantify some of the cost benefits of AT, Andrich developed the Siva Cost Analysis Instrument (SCAI).[1] This instrument assists in detailing or comparing the costs of various interventions. The tool can be used to guide economic considerations when choosing devices, to estimate and compare costs of options, or to calculate precisely the relative costs of interventions. The first step in this process is to itemize the following: (1) the overall objectives of the system, (2) foreseen evolution in case the system was not provided, (3) foreseen outcomes at the level of individual goals/expectations, (4) foreseen outcomes at the level of family expectations, (5) foreseen outcomes at the level of professional expectations, and (6) foreseen outcomes at the level of community expectations.[1]

The second stage of the process is to state the problem and list meaningful alternative options. The user and professional's preferences are then identified and the final choice noted. Time parameters are then defined.[1] Firstly, the time span of the program is noted, for example, how long the costs are to be monitored. Secondly, the period over which the solution is likely to remain meaningful is estimated for each intervention. Finally, the technical duration of each solution is determined. Andrich recommends that sophisticated computer technologies be costed over a 2- to 5-year period, whereas low-tech devices could be costed over 10 years.[1]

The final step in the SCAI process is to estimate the overall social cost and anticipated expenditure by the user, service provider, and others for purchase, maintenance, services, and assistance over the defined period of the solution. The tool is relatively easy to use; however, a day of training is recommended for effective use. One of the limitations noted by the developer is that estimates of duration and man-hours of assistance are based on assumptions that may vary between individuals; however, the author proposes that these assumptions do not affect the final output, which is primarily an economic comparison between options.[1] This tool allows comparison to be made between technologic and nontechnologic options, which is useful in comparing the actual cost of informal support. It provides a useful structure for anticipating the relative benefits of interventions, as well as the actual costs and benefits of a range of interventions. In a long-term retrospective study, Andrich, Ferrario, and Moi used the SCAI to examine the cost effectiveness of various interventions.[3] They noted that, when using the SCAI, the longer the time over which interventions are compared, the more likely it is that estimation errors will occur.[3] This tool is considered to be a "significant template for future cost analyses in AT" (p. 25).[40]

Participation

Following the introduction of the International Classification of Functioning, Disability, and Health (ICF),[106] service providers have developed an interest in whether interventions enable people to engage in activities and participate in community life. To date, workplace participation has been determined in terms of being employed or not employed,[70] being employed continuously for a specified period (e.g., the 12 weeks required by payers), or by comparing the amount of time employed with time available for employment.[61] Some studies have also examined the nature of work AT users undertake[30]; however, the quality of workplace participation has not yet been examined in detail, and standardized tools for evaluating workplace participation have not yet been developed. Although service providers, employers, and employees using AT are likely to be most interested in participation in employment-related activities and roles, assistive devices are frequently used across many activities and are likely to affect various aspects of life.

It has been proposed that the ICF provides a sound foundation for examining the impact of interventions on activity engagement and participation.[80,86] The ICF provides a checklist of activities,[105] including learning and applying knowledge; general tasks and demands; communication; mobility; self-care; domestic life; interpersonal relationships; major life areas, such as work; and community, social, and civic life, which allows a person's capacity and performance across many performance areas to be evaluated. Capacity evaluates the person's ability to execute the task without the assistance of another person, assistive device, or environmental modification. The performance qualifier measures the difficulty the person experiences in doing things, assuming that they want to do them. The scores range from 0 to 4, with 0 being no difficulty in performance or capacity and 4 being complete difficulty, which means a problem is present more than 95% of the time, with an intensity that totally disrupts the person's day-to-day life and that has happened every day over the last 30 days.[105] This checklist could be used to compare the person's general level of activity engagement and participation with and without assistive devices.[79]

Evaluation tools have also been developed that measure the quality of activity engagement and level of participation in various aspects of community life. Global tools such as OTFACT[93] and the Assessment of Life Habits (LIFE-H)[63] examine people's level of engagement in an extensive range of activities and participation across life areas. It is also expected that measures of participation, such as the Impact of Participation and Autonomy Questionnaire (IPAQ)[10] and the Participation Objective, Participation Subjective (POPS)[8] will continue to develop.

OTFACT, a software-based data collection system, enables service providers to record performance in a range of activities. This tool is multidimensional and uses Trichotomous Tailored Sub-branching Scaling (TTSS) to allow the question set to be customized to the specific needs of the AT user. As performance deficits are registered in an area, the software branches out, breaking down the activity into subsections so that discrete aspects of the performance can be examined in greater detail.[93] A percentage score is then calculated for activities relevant to the individual in which they are not able to participate fully. This is one of the few tools that provides a method for isolating the effect of AT.[79] OT FACT allows items to be scored under a range of conditions including with or without the use of AT. Scores obtained when using AT can then be directly compared to scores obtained without the use of AT.[79] The activity set in this tool is currently under revision, with a view to incorporating performance areas identified in the ICF. The TTSS system provides a good foundation for the development of customized scales to examine specific work activities in greater detail.

The LIFE-H is a questionnaire that is available in two forms. One is a screening tool (69 items) to identify areas of life in which participation in limited, and the other is an in-depth assessment (240 items) for examining participation across 12 domains.[63] The domains examined include nutrition, fitness, personal care, communication, residence, mobility, responsibility, interpersonal relations, community, education, employment, and recreation. The tool can be used by an external assessor or as a self-report tool to identify the level of difficulty experienced (and assistance required) by an individual in each area and for each activity on a 10-point scale.[63] The person's level of satisfaction with each life habit is also rated on a 5-point scale. Items that are not relevant to the person's life can be marked as not applicable.[63] The LIFE-H has been used to evaluate participation in people with a range of impairments, including cerebral palsy,[32,55,60] spinal cord injury,[64] and stroke,[23,25,26,75] as well as older adults.[24,62] Noreau, Fougeyrollas, and Vincent report that although the LIFE-H also has been used to evaluate the effect of environmental control systems, its use as an outcome measure for AT is limited.[63] This tool has been modified for working with children by excluding domains such as work, sexual relationships, and parenting roles. This indicates that this tool has the potential to be used for other applications, such as evaluating the participation of adults within the work environment.

Other measures of participation have been developed more recently, including the IPAQ[10] and the POPS,[8] which may prove to be useful in examining the impact of AT on participation in the future. The IPAQ is a 39-item questionnaire that examines an individual's perceived participation in a range of domains and perceived problem in each domain. Perceived participation is rated on a 5-point scale, with 1 being very good and 5 being very poor, in domains such as autonomy indoors and outdoors, family role, social situations, and paid work and education.[10] Perceived problems are rated from being no problem (= 0) to a severe problem (= 2). To date the IPAQ has been used to examine participation and perceived problems of people with spinal cord injuries[56] but has not been used to examine the impact of AT.

The POPS is a 26-item instrument that examines the societal/normative ("outsider") perspective and "insider perspective" of participation.[8] The PO (objective measures) examines the frequency or duration of engagement in activity in real-life environments, whereas the PS (subjective measures) examines the individual's satisfaction with his or her level of engagement in each activity, weighted by his or her rating of the activity's importance.[8] As a measure of both objective and subjective perspectives of participation, the POPS shows great promise.[56]

■ EVALUATING OUTCOME MEASURES

Given the preceding discussion of various AT outcome measures, it is worth reflecting on the parameters against which service providers evaluate the utility and integrity of these tools. In addition to the utility and integrity of measures, it is also critical to acknowledge what they fail to measure. Using any of these measures in isolation may attribute greater importance to some factors while others (which may be more difficult to capture) are disregarded, as reinforced by Albert Einstein in the opening quote of this chapter.

Although the AT industry has recently focused on developing suitable outcome measures, still only a limited number of suitable outcome measures are available.[20,22,33,56,85,92] Each of these tools, which rely on user feedback, has been designed to examine a specific aspect of AT outcomes, such as goal attainment, user satisfaction, well-being, and cost effectiveness. One of the most difficult aspects of evaluating the effectiveness of an intervention is deciding at the outset on suitable measures.[33] Stineman[95] proposed that seven factors should be considered when selecting an outcome measure:

- Breadth and depth (generalizability and specificity)
- Assessment and vantage point
- Objectivity
- Validity
- Reliability
- Responsiveness to change
- Method of scaling

Each of these will be discussed in turn as they relate to evaluating AT outcomes.

Global measures, that is, tools with breadth, will be applicable to a wide range of interventions and sample a broad spectrum of parameters, but depth is sacrificed when using global measures.[95] It is often difficult when using global tools, such as quality-of-life measures, to isolate the outcome to a specific intervention as the measure is likely to be influenced by a broad range of factors. In-depth tools, on the other hand, provide more specific information, which is often required to determine whether, and why, a device is meeting specific requirements. Although a number of generic tools are available that have been constructed to examine specific qualities of a defined number of devices, such as wheelchairs or computers,[95] there are few standardized tools that can be used to evaluate the relative benefit of these technologies.

Tools can also gather information from various vantage points.[95] For example, some seek information from consumers, whereas others are designed to be completed by clinicians. Both perspectives are critical for evaluating the effectiveness of AT interventions. Consumers are the only ones who can evaluate how well devices fit their personal preferences and working style and provide feedback on how well the device works for them in situ over time. Service providers, on the other hand, are often well placed to provide an outsider's perspective. They are often in a good position to provide users with insights into the consequences of, and potential barriers to, long-term device use and can select the appropriate AT outcomes measure to provide valuable information as required.

These tools can be used to assist both consumers and service providers in evaluating the relative advantages of solutions and to determine if the solution is able to maintain adequate performance over time. In the workplace environment, employers and supervisors also would have expectations of performance. Whether explicit or unspoken, these expectations need to be considered when evaluating the effectiveness of technology in enabling the AT user in the workplace.

Objective measures require information to be recorded in a standardized way, whereas subjective or self-report measures allow for personal responses to fixed response and open-ended questions.[95] Objective measures may include formal testing, direct observation of posture, rate, or duration of performance by a service provider, or records of errors, down-time, or work days lost. Subjective measures incorporate interviews, self-report questionnaires, or ratings. It is well recognized that both objective and subjective measures of AT quality and outcomes are required.[22] Traditionally, objective measures have been used by service providers to define the consumer's level of function and evaluate the fit and performance of the device. These measures can also be valuable to consumers, as they can provide accurate feedback on the person-technology and activity-technology fit. In particular, these tools can help consumers appreciate the functional benefits of specific options, compare the performance of options, and evaluate the ongoing effectiveness of their AT. Providing consumers with mechanisms to gather objective information on the performance of options empowers them to evaluate the functional value of options for themselves, rather than being dependent on service providers to make recommendations. This makes the process of determining the solution that best fits with the requirements of the person and tasks more transparent and allows the user to weigh the performance gains against other considerations, such as ease of use, to determine the hassle factor.[94] On the other hand, subjective or self-rated measures recognize the user's perspective and provide a mechanism to understand the user's experience of the technology. These tools are invaluable in evaluating the effectiveness of technology in the real world.

The psychometric properties of outcomes measures, that is, the validity and reliability of the measures, are important when considering the credibility of the evaluation process.[80] The quality of the measurement tools used has an impact on the quality of the data obtained.[38] In a recent review of outcomes measures used in AT outcomes studies, very few studies were found to report on the validity and reliability of the measures used.[54] Beyond measures focusing on AT specifically, valid and reliable rehabilitation and health outcome measures are available, but a recent review of 100 measures found that they varied widely in terms of the way AT was addressed in their scoring.[79] AT was incorporated into the outcome in only 22% of the tools examined and was ignored in the scoring of 30% of these tools, and actually lowered the functional score in 44% of the measures.[79] Tools that do not adequately document the use of AT in performance will result in reliability problems when service providers do not consistently acknowledge the consumer's use of AT.[79] Without a suitable conceptual or theoretical foundation that acknowledges the contribution of AT toward rehabilitation outcomes, evaluation tools will lack the construct validity required to measure AT outcomes, and more broad rehabilitation outcomes, effectively.[79]

Tools that are responsive to change are able to register behavior or outcomes as they improve or deteriorate.[95] These tools allow measures to be taken at various intervals, such as before and after intervention, or to compare outcomes immediately after purchase and at a review in the subsequent 6 or 12 months. This requires that tools are sensitive enough to be able to detect significant variation and have sufficient scope so that floor or ceiling effects are not created.[80] General purpose rehabilitation measures, such as the Functional Independence Measure (FIM),[98] have become benchmarks in terms of their psychometric properties; however, as noted previously, they are not very responsive to the impact of the use of a specific device.[33] The scoring in these tools does not reliably account for the impact of AT use, let alone provide sufficient sensitivity to measure changes in performance resulting from the use of a device. To be responsive, tools need to examine the quality of performance resulting from the AT user so that anticipated changes can be detected. This is particularly important for comparing the effectiveness of different AT solutions.

Finally, outcome measures vary in their use of measurement scales. The nature of the scaling method has implications for its meaningfulness and usability and sensitivity to change. For example, although rating pain (during the use of an AT device at work) on a scale of 1 to 100 may be sensitive to change for an individual, it is difficult to use such measures across consumers because of the subjective interpretation of pain in terms of absolute numbers. Service providers need to be cognizant of all these factors when selecting the most appropriate AT outcomes measures to evaluate the effectiveness of AT in the workplace.

SUMMARY

Clearly AT outcome evaluation is in its early stages of development. Given the limitations of the current tools, service providers need to take great care when selecting and using AT outcome measures. An important starting point is to establish the purpose of the evaluation and to ensure that the outcome measurement is consumer-centered. Care should be taken to ensure that the fit between the technology and the person, the activities, and the application environment(s) are all adequately evaluated. When choosing tools to assist in the evaluation process, service providers need to address the breadth and depth of the AT system, acknowledge the vantage point of the tool and examine the psychometric properties and measurement scale of the tool carefully. Evaluations should also be viewed in terms of how they can assist AT users to select and use technology effectively and be used throughout the process, as illustrated in this book, to assist users in evaluating the relative benefits of intervention options. The effective use of evaluation tools makes the process of selecting and evaluating options transparent and enables the user to have control over decisions and actively participate in the process. In addition, when used periodically to reevaluate the chosen device, these tools can assist users in identifying when the device is no longer adequately meeting their requirements. Consumers can then use this information to request a review of their AT system and explore suitable upgrades or alternatives. Throughout this book the need to recognize the ongoing cyclical nature of the AT process, which continues throughout the AT users' working life, has been highlighted. Regular evaluation allows consumers to progress smoothly through each cycle as each new device is investigated, trialed, funded, customized, and integrated into the work environment.

References

1. Andrich R: The SCAI instrument: measuring costs of individual assistive technology programs. *Technol Disabil* 14:95-99, 2002.
2. Andrich R, Besio S: Being informed, demanding and responsible consumers of assistive technology: an educational issue. *Disabil Rehabil* 24(1-3):152-159, 2002.
3. Andrich R, Ferrario M, Moi M: A model of cost-outcome analysis for assistive technology. *Disabil Rehabil* 20:1-24, 1998.
4. Batavia AI, Hammer GS: Toward the development of consumer-based criteria for the evaluation of assistive devices. *J Rehabil Res Development* 27(4):425-436, 1990.
5. Benedict RE, Lee JP, Marrujo SK, et al: Assistive devices as an early childhood intervention: evaluating outcomes. *Technol Disabil* 11:79-90, 1999.
6. Bottos M, Bocati C, Sciuto L, et al: Powered wheelchairs and independence in young children with tetraplegia. *Developmental Med Child Neurol* 43:769-777, 2001.
7. Brooks NA: Models for understanding rehabilitation and assistive technology, in Gray DB, Quatrano LA, Lieberman ML (eds): *Designing and Using Assistive Technology: The Human Perspective*. Baltimore, Paul H. Brookes, 1998.
8. Brown M, Dijkers M, Gordon WA, et al: Participation objective, participation subjective: a measure of participation combining outsider and insider perspectives. *J Head Trauma Rehabil* 19(6):459-481, 2004.
9. Buning ME, Angelo JA, Schmeler MR: Occupational performance and the transition to powered mobility: a pilot study. *Am J Occup Ther* 55(3):339-344, 2001.
10. Cardol M, de Haan RJ, de Jonge BA, et al: Psychometric properties of the Impact on Participation and Autonomy Questionnaire. *Arch Phys Med Rehabil* 82:210-216, 2004.
11. Carswell A, McColl MA, Baptiste S, et al: The Canadian Occupational Performance Measure: a research and clinical literature review. *Can J Occup Ther* 71(4):210-222, 2004.
12. Clemmer J: *Pathways to performance: a guide to transforming yourself, your team, and your organization*. Toronto, Macmillan Canada, 1995.
13. Cook A, Hussey S: *Assistive technologies: principles and practice*, ed 2. St. Louis, Mosby, 2002.
14. Cowan D, Turner-Smith A: The user's perspective on the provision of electronic assistive technology: equipped for life? *Br J Occup Ther* 62(1):2-6, 1999.
15. Cushman LA, Scherer MJ: Measuring the relationship of assistive technology use, functional status over time, and consumer-therapist perceptions of ATs. *Assistive Technol* 8:103-109, 1996.
16. Day H, Jutai JW: Measuring the psychosocial impact on assistive devices: the PAIDS. *Can J Rehabil* 9:159-168, 1996.
17. Dedding C, Cardol M, Eyssen IC, et al: Validity of the Canadian Occupational Performance Measure: a client-centered outcome measurement. *Clin Rehabil* 18(6):660-667, 2004.

18. Demers L, Weiss-Lambrou R, Ska B: Development of the Quebec User Evaluation of Satisfaction with Assistive Technology (QUEST). *Assistive Technol* 8:3-13, 1996.

19. Demers L, Weiss-Lambrou R, Ska B: The Quebec User Evaluation of Satisfaction with Assistive Technology (QUEST2.0): an overview and recent progress. *Technol Disabil* 14:101-105, 2002.

20. DeRuyter F: Evaluating outcomes in assistive technology: do we understand the commitment? *Assistive Technol* 7:3-16, 1995.

21. DeRuyter F: Outcomes and performance monitoring, in Olson DA, DeRuyter F (eds): *Clinician's Guide to Assistive Technology*. St. Louis, Mosby, 2001.

22. DeRuyter F: The importance of outcome measures for assistive technology service delivery systems. *Technol Disabil* 6:89-104, 1997.

23. Desrosiers J, Malouin F, Bourbonnais D, et al: Arm and leg impairments and disabilities after stroke rehabilitation: relation to handicap. *Clin Rehabil* 17(6):666-673, 2003.

24. Desrosiers J, Noreau L, Rochette A: Social participation of older adults in Quebec. *Aging Clin Experimental Res* 16(5):406-412, 2004.

25. Desrosiers J, Noreau L, Rochette A, et al: Predictors of handicap situations following post-stroke rehabilitation. *Disabil Rehabil* 24(15):774-785, 2002.

26. Desrosiers J, Rochette A, Noreau L, et al: Comparison of two functional independence scales with a participation measure in post-stroke rehabilitation. *Arch Gerontol Geriatrics* 37(2):157-172, 2003.

27. Donnelly C, Carswell A: Individualized outcome measures: a review of the literature. *Can J Occup Ther* 69(2):84-94, 2002.

28. Donnelly C, Eng JJ, Hall J, et al: Client-centered assessment and the identification of meaningful treatment goals for individuals with a spinal cord injury. *Spinal Cord* 42(5):302-307, 2004.

29. Douglas H, Swanson C, Gee T, et al: Outcome measurement in Australian rehabilitation environments. *J Rehabil Med* 37(5):325-329, 2005.

30. Dowler DL, Hirsh AE, Kittle RD, et al: Outcomes of reasonable accommodations in the workplace. *Technol Disabil* 5:345-354, 1996.

31. Enders A: *Technology for Life in a New Disability Paradigm. Keynote Presentation.* Paper presented at the Australian Conference on Technology for People with Disabilities, Sydney, September 28-30, 1999.

32. Fraser BA, Bryan D, Morano CK: Development of a physical characteristics assessment (PCA): a checklist for determining appropriate computer access for individuals with cerebral palsy. *Assistive Technol* 7:26-35, 1995.

33. Fuhrer MJ: Assistive technology outcomes research: challenges met and yet unmet. *Am J Phys Med Rehabil* 80(7):528-535, 2001.

34. Fuhrer MJ, Demers L, Scherer MJ, et al: Toward a taxonomy of assistive technology device outcomes. *Am J Phys Med Rehabil* 84(4):294-302, 2005.

35. Fuhrer MJ, Jutai JW, Scherer MJ, et al: A framework for the conceptual modeling of assistive technology device outcomes. *Disabil Rehabil* 25(22):1243-1251, 2003.

36. Galvin JC, Donnell CM: Educating the consumer and caretaker on assistive technology, in Scherer MJ (ed): *Assistive Technology: Matching Device and Consumer for Successful Rehabilitation*. Washington DC, American Psychological Association, 2002.

37. Garber S, Gregorio T: Upper extremity assistive devices: assessment of use by spinal cord injured patients with quadriplegia. *Am J Occup Ther* 44(2):126-131, 1990.

38. Gelderblom GJ, De Witte L: The assessment of assistive technology outcomes, effects and cost. *Technol and Disabil* 14:91-94, 2002.

39. Haigh R, Tennant A, Biering-Sorenson F, et al: The use of outcome measures in physical medicine and rehabilitation within Europe. *J Rehabil Med* 33(6):273-278, 2001.

40. Harris F, Sprigle S: Cost analyses in assistive technology research. *Assistive Technol* 15(1):16-27, 2003.

41. Heinemann AW: Measuring rehabilitation outcomes. *Technol Disabil* 12:129-143, 2000.

42. Hocking C: Function or feelings: factors in abandonment of assistive devices. *Technol Disabil* 11:3-11, 1999.

43. Jutai JW: Quality of life impact of assistive technology. *Rehabil Engineering* 14:2–7, 1999.

44. Jutai JW, Day H: Psychosocial Impact of Assistive Devices Scale (PIADS). *Technol Disabil* 14:107-111, 2002.

45. Jutai J, Day H, Woolrich W, et al: The predictability of retention and discontinuation of contact lenses. *Optometry* 74(5):299-308, 2003.

46. Jutai JW, Rigby P, Ryan S, et al: Psychosocial impact of electronic aids to daily living. *Assistive Technol* 12(2):123-131, 2000.

47. Keith RA: Patient satisfaction and rehabilitation services. *Arch Phys Med Rehabil* 79:1122-1128, 1998.

48. Kittel A, Di Marco A, Stewart H: Factors influencing the decision to abandon manual wheelchairs for three individuals with spinal cord injury. *Disabil Rehabil* 24(1-3):106-114, 2002.

49. Koester HH, LoPresti E, Ashlock G, et al: *Compass: software for computer skills assessment.* March 17-22, 2003. Retrieved November 12, 2005, from *http://www.csun.edu/cod/conf/2003/proceedings/165.htm.*

50. Law M: *Client-Centered Occupational Therapy.* Thorofare, NJ, SLACK Inc., 1998.

51. Law M, Baptiste S, Carswell A, et al: *Canadian Occupational Performance Measure,* ed 2. Toronto, Canadian Association of Occupational Therapists, 1994.

52. Lenker JA, Paquet VL: A new conceptual model for assistive technology outcomes research and practice. *Assistive Technol* 15:1-15, 2003.

53. Lenker JA, Paquet VL: A new conceptual model for assistive technology outcomes research and practice. *Assistive Technol* 16:1-10, 2004.

54. Lenker JA, Scherer MJ, Fuhrer MJ, et al: Psychometric and administrative properties of measures used in assistive technology device outcomes research. *Assistive Technol* 17(1):7-22, 2005.

55. Lepage C, Noreau L, Bernard PM, et al: Profile of handicap situations in children with cerebral palsy. *Scandinavian J Rehabil Med* 30(4):263-272, 1998.

56. Lund ML, Nordlund A, Nygard L, et al: Perceptions of participation and predictors of perceived problems with participation in persons with spinal cord injury. *J Rehabil Med* 37(1):3-8, 2005.

57. Malec JF: Goal attainment scaling in rehabilitation. *Neuropsychol Rehabil* 9(3-4):253-275, 1999.

58. Mann WC, Hurren D, Tomita M: Comparison of assistive device use and needs of home-based older persons with different impairments. *Am J Occup Ther* 47(11):980-987, 1993.

59. Mann WC, Tomita M: Perspectives on assistive devices among elderly persons with disabilities. *Technol Disabil* 9:119-148, 1998.

60. Morris C, Kurinczuk JJ, Fitzpatrick R: Child- or family-assessed measures of activity performance and participation for children with cerebral palsy: a structured review. *Child Care Health Development* 31(4):397-407, 2005.

61. Murphy GC, Young AE: Employment participation following spinal cord injury: relation to selected participant demographic, injury and psychological characteristics. *Disabil Rehabil* 27(21):1297-1306, 2005.

62. Noreau L, Desrosiers J, Robichaud L, et al: Measuring social participation: reliability of the LIFE-H in older adults with disabilities. *Disabil Rehabil* 26(6):346-352, 2004.

63. Noreau L, Fougeyrollas P, Vincent C: The LIFE-H: Assessment of the quality of social participation. *Technol Disabil* 14:113-118, 2002.

64. Norton K, Fougeyrollas P: Profile of social consequences of long-standing spinal injury: the occurrence of handicap situations. *Disabil Rehabil* 22(4):170-180, 2000.

65. Pape TLB, Kim J, Weiner B: The shaping of individual meanings assigned to assistive technology: a review of personal factors. *Disabil Rehabil* 24(1-3):5-20, 2002.

66. Patterson DR, Jensen M, Engel-Knowles J: Pain and its influence on assistive technology use, in Scherer MJ (ed): *Assistive Technology: Matching Device and Consumer for Successful Rehabilitation.* Washington DC, American Psychological Association, 2002.

67. Petty IS, Treviranus J: *Outcome Measures for High Technology Vision Aids: An Application of the Canadian Occupational Performance Measure,* 2003. Retrieved December 22, 2005, from *www.utoronto.ca/atrc/reference/atoutcomes/visionquest.html.*

68. Phillips B: Technology abandonment from the consumer point of view. *NARIC Quarterly* 3(2-3):4-91, 1993.

69. Phillips B, Zhao H: Predictors of assistive technology abandonment. *Assistive Technol* 5:36-45, 1993.

70. Pilling DS: Early employment careers of people with disabilities in the National Child Development Study. *Work* 18:75-87, 2002.

71. Post KM: The promise of assistive technology. *Am J Occup Ther* 47(11):965-967, 1993.

72. Poulson D, Richardson S: USERfit: a framework for user centered design in Assistive Technology. *Technol Disabil* 9:163-171, 1998.

73. Reimer-Reiss ML, Wacker RR: Factors associated with assistive technology discontinuance among individuals with disabilities. *J Rehabil* 66(3):44-50, 2000.

74. Ripat J, Booth A: Characteristics of assistive technology service delivery models: stakeholder perspectives and preferences. *Disabil Rehabil* 27(24):1461-1470, 2005.

75. Rochette A, Desrosiers J: Coping with the consequences of a stroke. *Int J Rehabil Res* 25(1):17-24, 2002.

76. Rodger S, de Jonge D, Fitzgibbon H: *Identifying Factors for Successful Integration of Persons with Disabilities Using Technology in the Workplace.* Canberra, Australia, Report to Commonwealth Department of Health and Family Services, 1999.

77. Rogers EM: *Diffusion of Innovations.* New York, Simon & Schuster, 1995.

78. Rushton PW, Miller WC: Goal attainment scaling in the rehabilitation of patients with lower-extremity amputations: a pilot study. *Arch Phys Med Rehabil* 83(6):771-775, 2002.

79. Rust KL, Smith RO: Assistive technology in the measurement of rehabilitation and health outcomes. *Am J Phys Med Rehabil* 84(10):780-793, 2005.

80. Salter K, Jutai JW, Teasell R, et al: Issues for selection of outcome measures in stroke rehabilitation: ICF body functions. *Disabil Rehabil* 27(4):191-207, 2005.

81. Saunders GH, Jutai JW: Hearing specific and generic measures of the psychosocial impact of hearing aids. *J Am Acad Audiol* 15(3):238-248, 2004.

82. Scherer MJ: Assessing technology use, avoidance and abandonment: What we know so far. *Proceedings of the Sixth Annual Conference on Technology and Persons with Disabilities* (pp. 815–826), California State University, Northridge, 1991.

83. Scherer MJ: *Living in a State of Stuck: How Assistive Technology Impacts the Lives of People with Disabilities*, ed 4. Cambridge, Mass, Brookline Books, 2005.
84. Scherer MJ: The impact of assistive technology on the lives of people with disabilities, in Gray DB, Quatrano LA, Lieberman ML (eds): *Designing and Using Assistive Technology: The Human Perspective*. Baltimore, Paul H. Brookes, 1998.
85. Scherer MJ: *The Matching Person & Technology (MPT) Model Manual and Assessment*, ed 5, [CD-ROM]. Webster, NY, The Institute for Matching Person & Technology, Inc., 2005.
86. Scherer MJ, Glueckauf R: Assessing the benefits of assistive technologies for activities and participation. *Rehabil Psychol* 50(2):132-141, 2005.
87. Scherer MJ, Sax CL, Vanbiervliet A, et al: Predictors of assistive technology use: the importance of personal and psychosocial factors. *Disabil Rehabil* 27(21):1321-1331, 2005.
88. Schlosser RW: Goal Attainment Scaling as a clinical measurement technique in communication disorders: a critical review. *J Commun Disord* 37(3):217-239, 2004.
89. Schwanke TD, Smith RO: Assistive technology outcomes in work settings. *Work* 24:195-204, 2005.
90. Siggeirsdottir K, Alfredsdottir U, Einarsdottir G, et al: A new approach in vocational rehabilitation in Iceland: preliminary report. *Work* 22(1):3-8, 2004.
91. Smith RO: IMPACT 2 Model, 2005. Retrieved December 12, 2005, from *http://www.uwm.edu/CHS/r2d2/archive/impact2model.html*.
92. Smith RO: Measuring the outcomes of assistive technology: challenge and innovation, *Assist Technol* 8:71-81, 1996.
93. Smith RO: OTFACT: multi-level performance-oriented software assistive technology outcomes protocol. *Technol Disabil* 14:133-139, 2002.
94. Sprigle S, Abdelhamied A: The relationship between ability measures and assistive technology selection, design and use, in Gray DB, Quatrano LA, Lieberman ML (eds): *Designing and Using Assistive Technology: The Human Perspective*. Baltimore, Paul H. Brookes, 1998.
95. Stineman MG: The spheres of self-fulfillment: a multidimensional approach to the assessment of assistive technology outcomes, in Gray DB, Quatrano LA, Lieberman ML (eds): *Designing and Using Assistive Technology: The Human Perspective*. Baltimore, Paul H Brookes, 1998.
96. Strong G, Jutai JW, Bevers P, et al: The psychosocial impact of closed-circuit television (CCTV) low vision aids. *Visual Impairment Res* 5(3), 2004.
97. Tam C, Reid D, Naumann S, O'Keefe B: Perceived benefits of word prediction intervention on written productivity in children with spina bifida and hydrocephalus. *Occup Ther Int* 9:237-255, 2002.
98. Uniform Data System for Medical Rehabilitation (UDS): *Functional Independence Measure*, Version 5.1. Buffalo, NY, Buffalo General Hospital, State University of New York, 1997.
99. Vanbiervliet A, Parette HP: Development and evaluation of the families, cultures and Augmentative and Alternative Communication (ACC) multimedia program. *Disabil Rehabil* 24(1-3):131-143, 2002.
100. Weiss-Lambrou R: Satisfaction and comfort, in Scherer MJ (ed): *Assistive Technology: Matching Device and Consumer for Successful Rehabilitation*. Washington DC, American Psychological Association, 2002.
101. Wessels RD, De Witte LP, Jedeloo S, et al: Effectiveness of provision of outdoor mobility services and devices in the Netherlands. *Clin Rehabil* 18:371-378, 2004.

102. Wessels R, Persson J, Lorentsen O, et al: IPPA: Individually Prioritised Problem Assessment. *Technol Disabil* 14:141-145, 2002.
103. Wessels RD, Willems CG, de Witte LP: How to select a method to evaluate usability of assistive devices. *J Rehabil Sci* 9(2):53-57, 1996.
104. Wielandt PM, McKenna K, Tooth LR, et al: Post discharge use of bathing equipment prescribed by occupational therapists: what lessons to be learned? *Phys Occup Ther Geriatrics* 19(3):49-65, 2001.
105. World Health Organization: *ICF Checklist*, 2005. Retrieved January 20 2005, from *www3.who.int/icf/checklist/icf-checklist.pdf.*
106. World Health Organization: International Classification of Function, Disability and Health: ICF, Geneva, WHO, 2001.

Questions to Guide Identifying Potential Technologies

▨ VISIONING POSSIBILITIES

1. Do I understand what technology can offer me? Now? In the future?
2. Do I know about services/resources that can assist me in exploring technology possibilities?
   - Colleagues with similar needs
   - AT user
   - Computer-literate friends/relatives
   - Disability organizations/support groups
   - AT services
   - Rehabilitation counselors
   - IT personnel
   - Human resources personnel
   - Computer/technology publications
   - Internet sites and databases
   - Technology manufacturers/suppliers
   - Employer/coworkers
3. Have I had a chance to see someone using suitable/potential technologies?
4. Have I talked with them about the benefits/limitations of these technologies?
   Before progressing to the next step:
   1. Do I understand how technology might assist me?
   2. Am I confident that technology has something to offer me?

▨ AWARENESS OF NEEDS

Analyze current method
1. Am I working efficiently using my current methods?
2. Am I experiencing unnecessary discomfort or pain?
3. Have I discussed my difficulties with anyone?
   Define needs and technology requirements
4. What tasks does/will my job entail?
5. What tasks am I experiencing/likely to experience difficulty with?
6. What aspect of the task/s is proving/likely to prove most problematic?
7. Can these tasks be reassigned or modified?
8. Am I aware of any technologies that could assist with these tasks?

9. Create a list of the things you would like technology to be able to do.

_____

_____

_____

_____

_____

_____

_____

10. Have you had previous experience with technology? What have these experiences told you about how your preferences and skills are related to using and managing technology? Consider the following:
    - Complexity of technology
    - Look/aesthetics of the device
    - Portability
    - Reliability/durability
    - Ease of use
    - Comfort with use
    - Training requirements
    - Flexibility
    - Comfort
    - Adjustability
    - Compatibility
    - Support requirements

11. Does/will the working environment have any specific requirements of the technology? Consider the following:
    - Location/s technology to be used
    - Workspace available
    - Shared workspace/technologies
    - Noise/sound/light constraints
    - Productivity expectations
    - Existing computer infrastructure/network
    - Availability of learning support
    - Availability of maintenance and repair
    - Availability of upgrades

12. Do I have access to a service provider who can assist me with defining my needs?

13. What are my future needs likely to be? Am I likely to need these technologies in other workspaces? Am I likely to change jobs? Am I likely to need similar technologies in other locations (e.g., at home)? Are there other tasks I would like to be able to do with this technology?

14. Are these technologies likely to develop in the near future?
    Before progressing to the next step:
    Write down your specific needs and identify the characteristics these require of potential technologies.

Needs	Technology Requirements
Personal	
Tasks/Activities	
Environment	

◼ FIND OUT WHAT IS AVAILABLE

1. Have I listed my specific technology requirements?
2. Have I constructed a list of questions I need answered?
3. Have I explored my technology requirements with any of the following?
   - Colleagues with similar needs
   - AT users
   - Computer-literate friends/relatives
   - Disability organizations/support groups
   - Assistive technology services
   - Rehabilitation counselors
   - IT personnel
   - Human resources personnel
   - Technology manufacturers/suppliers
   - Employer/coworkers
4. Are these service/resources assisting me to address my specific needs? If not, are there other services/resources better suited to meeting my needs?
5. Have I allocated adequate time to explore my technology options?
   Before progressing to the next step:
   Am I confident that I know about the range of technology options that might be suited to my needs?

Questions to Guide Trialing Devices

1. Where can I trial each of these options?
2. Have I trialed each option?
3. Have I trialed the best of these in the work environment or to complete work tasks?
4. Do I understand the features of each device?
5. Was each device adjusted to meet my individual needs during the trial?
6. Was the trial long enough for me to evaluate long-term use of this device?
7. How well does each device meet each of my needs/technology requirements?
8. Evaluate the relative benefit of each device against your technology requirements. How well does each device meet each requirement?

TECHNOLOGY REQUIREMENTS	DEVICE 1	DEVICE 2	DEVICE 3
Person	1 2 3 4 5	1 2 3 4 5	1 2 3 4 5
Tasks	1 2 3 4 5	1 2 3 4 5	1 2 3 4 5
Environment	1 2 3 4 5	1 2 3 4 5	1 2 3 4 5

Key:

1   2   3   4   5

not at all——somewhat——very well

Additional questions to ask about each device:

9. Do I experience any discomfort or pain when using this device?
10. How efficiently can I work using this device?
11. Will it be difficult for me to use and maintain?
12. Will it work with other technologies I will be using?
13. Will it work well in my workplace?

Questions to Guide Choosing the Best Technology

1. Which technology requirements are most important?
2. Do the other stakeholders (e.g., my employer, rehabilitation counselor, AT service provider) understand all my needs?
3. Do I understand their perspective?
4. Which device meets my requirements best?
5. Is there a mainstream product with the same functionality?
6. Have I been able to direct this process?

   Before you make your final choice:
   - Do I feel that I have sufficient information on and experience of the devices to make an informed choice?
   - Am I confident in the final choice?

7. Consider reviewing technology needs when:
   - There are changes in my function or skills
   - The current technology becomes unreliable or stops functioning
   - Workplace technologies are being reviewed or upgraded
   - There have been further developments in my device or related technologies

Questions to Guide the Acquisition of Technology

1. Have I alerted people to my needs?
2. Have I enlisted the right people to assist me in identifying my technology needs?
3. Is my employer aware of my technology requirements?
4. Are any of the following likely to impact on having my needs met in a timely way?
   - Outdated technology in the workplace
   - Limited access to computers at work
   - Delays in the approval process
   - Device needs to be imported
   - Supplier delays
   - Installation delays
5. Are upgrades required to the existing platform technologies?
6. Have my technology requirements been forwarded to the relevant people?
7. Do I know where I can get funding for my technology?
   - Employer
   - Government
   - Tax incentives
   - Community groups
   - Interest-free loan
8. Will the funding allow me to take the technology to my next workplace?
9. Will the funding allow me to use the technology offsite/at home?
10. Will the funding be adequate to cover the following?
    - Upgrading of computer platform
    - Down time for training
    - Device/software training
    - IT support
    - Repairs and maintenance
    - Regular upgrading of device/software

Questions to Guide Choosing a Supplier

1. Does the supplier provide you with a clear understanding of how the device works?
2. Does the supplier provide you with a clear understanding of how the device can be used?
3. Does the supplier know how the device can be integrated with other systems?
4. Who is responsible for maintenance and service? Is there an easily understood service manual included? Does the dealer provide replacement equipment while the device is being serviced?
5. Has the system been field tested? What sort of formal evaluation has the device undergone? What are the relevant standards the device has to be tested against?
6. Does the supplier have an established relationship with the manufacturer of this product?
7. Can I upgrade this product as new features are developed? Is this an additional cost?
8. Does the supplier assist or support the installation and ongoing compatibility issues of the product? Is this incorporated into the overall cost or is it an extra cost?
9. Does the user or support person require training to set up or use this product? Where can it be obtained? What are the costs?

Questions to Guide Working with a Supplier

1. What type of products does this supplier distribute?
2. What range of brands does this supplier support?

▦ PRESENTATION OF INFORMATION

3. Does the supplier communicate in a way that is easy to understand?
4. Do I feel heard and understood? Are my questions answered?
5. Can I take away printed information?
6. Do I have a clear understanding of the product and what it can do?
7. Does the supplier refer to clients respectfully?

▦ CONTENT

8. Can the supplier provide me with a clear understanding of how the device works?
9. Can the supplier provide me with a clear understanding of how the device can be used?
10. Can the supplier demonstrate ways in which the device can be customized to suit my needs?
11. Can the supplier provide me with examples of ways in which this device is being used in a range of environments?
12. Does the supplier know how the device can be integrated with other systems?

▦ ONGOING SUPPORT

13. Does the supplier assist or support the installation and ongoing compatibility issues of the product? Is this incorporated into the overall cost or is it an extra cost?
14. Who is responsible for maintenance and service? Is an easily understood service manual included? Does the dealer provide replacement equipment while the device is being serviced?
15. Will I need training or support to set up or use this product? Where can it be obtained? What are the costs?

▓ INDUSTRY SUPPORT

16. Is the supplier aware of similar products? Do they supply any of them?
17. Can the supplier compare products to other similar products which they don't supply?
18. Has the system been field tested? What sort of formal evaluation has the device undergone? What are the relevant standards the device has to be tested against?
19. Does the supplier have an established relationship with the manufacturer of this product? How long have they been supplying this product?
20. Can I upgrade this product as new features are developed? Is this an additional cost?

Questions to Guide Customization

■ COMFORT

1. Do I feel any tension, fatigue, or pain while using this device? Where do I feel this tension/fatigue?
2. Have I talked with someone about the tension, fatigue, or pain I am experiencing? If so, have I recorded:
   - *When* I experience discomfort
   - *Where* I experience the discomfort
   - *What* I am doing at the time I experience discomfort
   - If it intensifies or happens more quickly over time
3. Am I holding an awkward or unsupported posture for a long period?
4. Am I using an awkward movement repeatedly?
5. Do I perform any movements that I find particularly effortful?
6. Am I likely to be using these movements for many years?
7. Am I working efficiently?
8. Am I working as quickly as required?
9. Am I able to change position and vary my movements periodically?
10. Am I able to take regular rest breaks?
11. Am I positioned ergonomically (e.g., joints in a neutral position, head in alignment)?

■ WORK POSITION

12. Is my seating comfortable?
13. Does it allow me to maintain an active sitting posture (sit upright and work comfortably)?
14. Am I adequately supported by the seat and back rest?
15. Is the keyboard/working surface at or slightly below elbow height?
16. Does the working surface limit the amount of flexion in my upper spine and neck?
17. Can I view the screen with my head in a neutral position?
18. Can my hands rest in a neutral position over the keyboard?
19. Am I able to comfortably reach all areas of the keyboard?
20. Are frequently used keys easily accessible? (Please visit the U.S. Department of Labor, Occupational Safety and Health Administration Web site for further information on ergonomic working postures at computer workstations *www.osha.gov/SLTC/etools/computerworkstations/components.html*).
21. Do I understand how to make adjustments to my seating, monitor, and keyboard position?

22. Are these adjustments easily undertaken?
23. Does my workstation allow me to position all my equipment ergonomically?
24. Do I take time to regularly adjust my workstation so that I maintain an ergonomic posture?
25. Do people comment on my working postures?
26. Do I need to access a service provider to assist me in achieving an ergonomic position?
27. Have I identified a date when I will review the ergonomics of my workstation again?

▓ EFFICIENCY

28. Are there shortcuts or macros I could be using to decrease the number of keystrokes I use?
29. Do I have alternative methods/technologies I can use to vary my working positions and movements?
30. Are other technologies available that would reduce effort and improve my efficiency?

Questions to Guide Learning to Use Your Technology

KNOWLEDGE OF THE TECHNOLOGY

1. Do I know all the features and functions of my technology?
2. Do I know how to use/adjust these? Have I consulted the help function or manual?
3. Do I know people who know about these features and functions? Consider asking or consulting the following people/resources:
   - Other AT users
   - Work colleagues
   - Computer-literate friends/relatives
   - Disability organizations/support groups
   - Assistive technology services
   - Rehabilitation counselors
   - IT personnel
   - Human resources personnel
   - Computer/technology publications
   - Internet sites and databases
   - Technology manufacturers/suppliers
   - Online tutorials
4. Have I made a time to ask them?
5. Have I identified a "circle of support" for customizing my technology?
6. Have I identified a time when I will regularly review my technology adjustments?

Note: How will I know when this technology is no longer meeting my needs?

ACCESS TO SUITABLE TRAINING

7. Have I allocated time to learn to use my technology?
8. Do I have access to these technologies out of work hours to become more familiar with them?
9. Once I have mastered the basics, will I have access to ongoing training resources?
10. Have I discussed my training requirements with my employer and rehabilitation/human resources officer?
11. Do they understand my ongoing training needs?
12. What methods do I find most helpful when learning about technology?
    - Step-by-step demonstration
    - Watching others

- Experimentation
- Trial and error
- Practice
- Reading the manual or Help screens
- Completing online tutorials

13. Have I accessed resources that can assist me in using my technology?
    - Other AT users
    - Work colleagues
    - Computer-literate friends/relatives
    - Disability organizations/support groups
    - Assistive technology services
    - Rehabilitation counselors
    - IT personnel
    - Human resources personnel
    - Computer/technology publications
    - Internet sites and databases
    - Technology manufacturers/suppliers
    - Online tutorials

14. Does the trainer understand:
    - My current skills and experience? Am I a novice, intermediate, or advanced user?
    - The tasks I am required to perform?
    - The existing demands and supports in the work environment?

15. Has the trainer developed training objectives with me?
16. Have the training objectives been stated explicitly?

◼ TRAINING EXPERIENCE

17. Does the trainer clearly outline the objectives of the training session?
18. Do these meet my training needs?
19. Do I understand what the technology does?
20. Do I know how to use this technology to complete work tasks?
21. Do I know how to perform specific functions related to my work?
22. Does the session allow me to practice what I have learned?
23. Have I developed skills in using the basic functions?
24. Do I know where to go to develop more advanced skills?
25. Do I know how to diagnose and fix problems?
26. Do I know how to find out about other functions?
27. Am I able to extend the capabilities of the technology to meet my specific needs?

Questions to Guide the Long-Term Use of Assistive Technology in the Workplace

1. Does my employer expect me to initiate requests for technology review?
2. Do I understand funding systems, my rights, legislation, and how to negotiate with my employer?
3. Can I justify the need for accommodations in language that the employer or funding body will understand?
4. Is there someone who can assist me with advocating for my technology needs in the workplace?
   - Other AT user
   - Work colleague/supervisor
   - Rehabilitation counselor
   - Advocacy group
   - Assistive technology service
   - IT personnel
   - Human resources personnel
   - Equal opportunity officer
5. Does my employer understand funding systems, legislation, and AT service systems?
6. Does my employer know who can assist him/her in addressing my technology requirements?
7. Is my workplace AT-user friendly?
   - Are my coworkers/employer(s) friendly and supportive?
   - Are they comfortable discussing my technology requirements?
   - Are they fair in negotiating my needs?
   - Do they accept that I have specific technology requirements?
   - Are antidiscrimination policies in place and actively followed?
   - Is there a clear process for identifying and dealing with accommodation issues?
   - Does the employer seek appropriate resources and expertise to assist with meeting my technology requirements?
   - Are they responsive to requests for technology review?
   - Do they anticipate the impact of changes in the workplace on my technology use?
   - Is there a process for regularly reviewing my technology needs?

Resources and Web Links

▤ FUNDING

Informed Consumer's Guide to Funding Assistive Technology
ABLEDATA
8630 Fenton Street, Suite 930
Silver Spring, MD 20910
800-227-0216
301-608-8998
301-608-8958 (fax)301-608-8912 (TT)
http://www.abledata.com/abledata_docs/funding.htm

▤ AT ASSOCIATIONS

Association for the Advancement of Assistive Technology in Europe (AAATE)
AAATE c/o Danish Centre Gregersensvej, Gate 38 DK-2630
Taastrup, Denmark
+45 43 52 70 72 (fax)
http://www.aaate.net/

Australian Rehabilitation and Assistive Technology Association (ARATA)
c/- Technical Solutions Pty Ltd
109 Ferndale
SILVAN VIC
Australia 3795
http://www.e-bility.com/arata/

Rehabilitation Engineering and Assistive Technology Society of North America (RESNA)
1700 N. Moore St., Suite 1540
Arlington, VA 22209-1903
703-524-6686
703-524-6630 (fax)
703-524-6639 (TTY)
http://www.resna.org/

Rehabilitation Engineering Society of Japan (RESJA)
c/o Laboratory of Adaptive and Assistive Engineering Department of Ecosystem Engineering, Graduate School of Engineering
The University of Tokushima
2-1 Minami-josajima-cho
Tokushima, 770-8506, Japan

+81 88 656 2167
+81 88 656 2168 (fax)
http://www.resja.gr.jp/eng/index.html

■ LISTSERVS FOR ASSISTIVE TECHNOLOGY USERS

Cat-1st
http://groups.yahoo.com/group/cat-1st
Jaws for Windows
http://www.wdev.net/oldjfw
Voice Users Mailing List
http://voicerecognition.com/voice-users/

■ PROFESSIONAL ORGANIZATIONS

American Counseling Association (ACA)
5999 Stevenson Ave
Alexandria, VA 22304
800-347-6647
800-473-2329 (fax)
703-823-6862 (TDD)
http://www.counseling.org/

American Occupational Therapy Association (AOTA)
4720 Montgomery Lane
PO Box 31220
Bethesda, MD 20824-1220
301-652-2682
301-652-7711 (fax)
1-800-377-8555 (TDD)
http://www.aota.org/

American Rehabilitation Counseling Association (ARCA)
5999 Stevenson Ave
Alexandria, VA 22304
800-347-6647
800-473-2329 (fax)
703-823-6862 (TDD)
http://www.arcaweb.org/

American Speech-Hearing Association (ASHA)
10801 Rockville Pike
Rockville, MD 20852
800-498-2071
301-571-0457 (fax)
301-897-5700 (TTY)
http://www.asha.org/default.htm

International Center for Disability Resources on the Internet (ICDRI)
5212 Covington Bend Drive
Raleigh, NC 27613
919-349-6661
http://www.icdri.org/

The National Business and Disability Council (NBDC)
201 I.U. Willets Road
Albertson, NY 11507
516-465-1515
516-465-3730 (fax)
http://www.business-disability.com/

National Counsel on Rehabilitation Education (NCRE)
Rehabilitation Counseling Program
Kremen School of Education & Human Development
California State University–Fresno
5005 N. Maple Ave, M/S ED 3
Fresno, CA 0740-8025
559-278-0325 559-278-0016 (fax)
http://www.rehabeducators.org/

National Employment Counseling Association (NECA)
5999 Stevenson Ave
Alexandria, VA 22304
800-347-6647
800-473-2329 (fax)
703-823-6862 (TDD)
http://employmentcounseling.burcopsg.net/neca.html

RESEARCH RESOURCES

Disability and Rehabilitation: Assistive Technology
www.tandf.co.uk/journals/titles/17483107.asp
The National Assistive Technology Advocacy Project
http://www.nls.org/natmain.htm
Assistive Technology
www.resna.org/ProfResources/Publications/ATJournal.php
Technology and Disability
www. iospress.nl/html/10554181.php

Index

Page numbers followed by *f, t,* and *b*
indicate figures, tables, and boxed
material, respectively.